Refugee Children

The last 20 years have seen unprecedented numbers of refugee children entering Western countries. Many of these children will have experienced the atrocities of war and issues concerning their care and treatment are high on the agenda of research bodies, policy makers and service providers.

Refugee Children is the first book to offer a wide-ranging analysis of the context of care and the measures taken by nation states and intergovernmental bodies to address perceived problems. Drawing on a detailed examination of practices, the book outlines a model of good practice in the care of refugee children. Topics covered include:

- the treatment of asylum-seeking children at the borders of industrialised countries
- reception, psycho-social problems, social capital, education, and issues relating to cultural diversity and integration
- a critical analysis of responses to these problems including the development of special programmes for refugee children
- elements of good practice in the field
- the transfer of good practice between countries
- implications for the development of services and academic research in this vital area.

With a series of case studies examining practices from a number of countries, *Refugee Children* makes a vital contribution both to the social care literature in this field and to theory and research in refugee and migration studies. As such it is essential reading for academic researchers in a range of disciplines including social policy, education, migration and refugee studies as well as service providers in health care, social care, housing and education.

Charles Watters is Director of the European Centre for the Study of Migration and Social Care in the School of Social Policy, Sociology and Social Research at the University of Kent.

Refugee Children
Towards the next horizon

Charles Watters

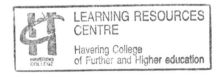
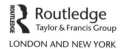

Routledge
Taylor & Francis Group

LONDON AND NEW YORK

First published 2008
by Routledge
2 Park Square, Milton Park, Abingdon, Oxon OX14 4RN

Simultaneously published in the USA and Canada
by Routledge
270 Madison Ave, New York, NY 10016

Routledge is an imprint of the Taylor & Francis Group, an informa business

© 2008 Charles Watters

Typeset in Times by
GreenGate Publishing Services, Tonbridge, Kent
Printed and bound in Great Britain by
Antony Rowe Ltd, Chippenham, Wilts

British Library Cataloguing in Publication Data
A catalogue record for this book is available from the British Library

Library of Congress Cataloging in Publication Data
Watters, Charles, 1956-
Refugee children : towards the next horizon / Charles Watters.
p. cm.
Includes bibliographical references and index.
1. Refugee children. 2. Refugee children--Services for. I. Title.
HV640.W337 2008
362.87--dc22
2007020940

ISBN-10: 0–415–38305–6 (hbk)
ISBN-10: 0–415–38306–4 (pbk)

ISBN-13: 978–0–415–38305–9 (hbk)
ISBN-13: 978–0–415–38306–6 (pbk)

Contents

1 Introduction

When I considered writing a book on refugee children, I was immediately confronted by questions concerning its scope and related questions regarding the definition of 'refugee children'. The more I engaged in research on the topic, the greater the potential areas of investigation became. One could easily argue that one book alone would be totally insufficient to address the issues affecting refugee children even in one country or region of the world. At the time of writing, the everyday brutality of the situations in Darfur, Somalia, Iraq and the Democratic Republic of Congo, to name a few, are giving rise to the forced displacement of thousands of people, many of them children, who cross international borders in the hope of protection. By the end of 2005, Afghanistan was by far the largest country of origin of refugees, with no less than 1.9 million Afghan refugees reported in 72 asylum countries (UNHCR, 2006a). All of these situations have a profound impact on children under the age of 18 who make up an estimated 44 per cent of the total population 'of concern' to United Nations High Commission for Refugees (UNHCR). The scale and complexity of the field is indicated further by the considerable regional variation in the proportion of children involved and the types of displacement experienced. Those recorded as being 'of concern' to UNHCR include refugees, asylum seekers, internally displaced persons and stateless persons. The proportion of children in this overall population of approximately 20.8 million at the end of 2005 (UNHCR, 2006a) varies considerably from region to region with 54 per cent aged under 18 in Africa, 46 per cent in Asia and 25 per cent in Europe (UNHCR, 2006b, p22).

As will be discussed below, these figures reflect different dynamics of displacement. As UNHCR notes, 'the vast majority of the world's refugee children seek sanctuary in poor countries' and have neither the resources nor the capacity to travel to wealthy industrialised countries (ibid.). In general, in the first decade of the new millennium, countries with mass refugee situations are those in the developing world and these also have proportionately higher numbers of refugee women and children among refugee populations. The gender and age balance differs considerably among those seeking asylum in 'developed' countries, with fewer children and a significantly higher proportion of males.

Besides geographical and numerical disparities, the subject matter immediately raises definitional issues. As Zolberg has noted, 'although the term *refugee* has deep historical roots, its significance as a legal and administrative category has been vastly enhanced in our own times' (Zolberg *et al.*, 1989, p3, emphasis in original). Along with this increase in significance, the category 'refugee' has been more narrowly defined within legal and administrative contexts. According to the Protocol Relating to the Status of Refugees agreed upon by the UN in 1967, the term has a very specific meaning applying to any person,

> who is outside the country of his nationality...because he has or had well-founded fear of persecution by reason of his race, religion, nationality, membership of a particular social group or political opinion and is unable or, because of such fear, is unwilling to avail himself of the protection of the government of the country of his nationality.
>
> (Ibid., p4)

As will be discussed below, the focus of this book is not restricted to legal and administrative definitions of refugee children based on the protocol, but instead accords with what Zolberg has referred to as a 'sociological' definition 'grounded in observable social realities' (1989, p4). As such, rather than taking its point of departure from legal definitions, the operation of these definitions 'on the ground' constitutes part of the field of enquiry. Accordingly, many of the children considered in the study will not be granted refugee status; some will be expelled from territories without having access to information or resources that would enable them to make an asylum claim, others will be placed in detention or reception centres while an asylum claim is considered, only for it to be rejected and the child deported. Indeed refugee status is accorded to a very small minority of children in industrialised countries owing to a prevailing 'culture of disbelief' while a significantly higher proportion are allowed to remain for limited periods on humanitarian grounds (Bhabha and Crock, 2007). Rather than being led by prevailing legal definitions, I use the term 'refugee children' in a capacious way to refer to children who are seeking refuge in industrialised countries owing to adverse circumstances in their countries of origin. Many of the children considered here make applications for asylum, but substantial numbers do not or cannot owing to various constraints arising from the policies of deterrence pursued by potential host countries.

My decision to focus the book on refugee children in industrialised countries is not therefore based on a prior calculation of numbers or of needs, but on a growing concern to understand a crisis on the 'doorstep' of the world's richest nations. The study is informed by accounts of refugee children's experiences, but its primary focus is not on presenting 'stories' of displaced people themselves, of which there are several good recent examples (Jones, 2004; Moorehead, 2005; Yaghmaian, 2005; Molano, 2005 to name a few). The focus instead is on what may broadly be described as the ways in which refugee children are *treated* when they seek to cross borders into the industrialised world. I argue that children find themselves at a number of interfaces between what may be described as technologies of government. These include concerns with security and territorial integrity or what may be called the '*immigration control trajectory*' and what I have described as the '*welfare trajectory*' which is oriented towards programmes of social support and, increasingly, psychosocial well-being. The interrelationship between these aspects of government reveals acute tensions between conflicting views of the refugee children as 'untrustworthy children' or as 'damaged children' requiring psychological and emotional rehabilitation.

The content and purpose of this typology is rather different to influential generic and sociological approaches suggested, for example, by James, Jenks and Prout (1998). In examining how the child is constituted sociologically, James *et al.* outline four orientations; the socially constructed child, the tribal child, the minority group child and the social-structural child (James *et al.*, 1998). The orientation of the present study is towards representing ideal typical forms generated through *practice* rather than through an overview of academic theories. I include an examination of a range of responses to refugee children, from border controls and age assessments to educational and psychosocial interventions. In doing so, I attempt to identify and examine salient discourses on refugee children that are embedded in a range of services and institutional responses.

My concern here is not only to examine the way in which industrialised countries respond to refugee children, but also to argue for a particular methodological orientation in examining these responses. It is proposed that a 'thin' description of various programmes offered in countries is insufficient as it tells us little about the social and political contexts in which such programmes arise and the professional discourses that underpin them. I argue instead for a multi-level 'thick' description in which programmes are examined in the context of macro-, meso- and micro-level aspects. I postulate that this approach is not only theoretically important but also necessary at a practical level if programmes are to be transferred successfully from region to region, country to country.

A further area of concern is the transformation of services themselves. Here I eschew casual distinctions between the world of academic research and the world of policy and practice. I argue that 'thick' analysis, far from being an academic indulgence, is here a prerequisite for meaningful and enduring change in services. As Turton has argued, 'the best way to make scientific knowledge "relevant" to practice is to use it to scrutinise and problematise what practical knowledge takes for granted, not to sustain or legitimise it' (Turton, 2003, p17). Turton draws on Castles' observations of the potential weakness of policy-driven research to support his argument:

> The key point is that policy-driven research can lead not only to poor sociology but also to bad policy. This is because narrowly focussed empirical research, often designed to provide an answer to an immediate bureaucratic problem, tends to follow a circular logic. It accepts the problem definitions built into its terms of reference, and does not look for more fundamental causes, nor for more challenging solutions.
>
> (Castles, 2003, p26)

The present study seeks to move away both from a narrowly policy-driven research focus and from scientific measures administered on the basis of a premise that refugee children have various problems that should be rectified. Rather, its focus is on examination of the ways in which refugee children come to be construed as 'problems' and the roles of professionalised discourses in postulating and analysing the nature of their problems.

I pay particular attention to the response of public services with responsibility for children's welfare and the plethora of special programmes that have been established in response to refugee children's perceived needs. My approach has not been to offer a country by country account of the treatment of refugee children, but to draw on examples from a range of countries to illustrate particular aspects of their treatment. In doing so, it is not my intention either to single out particular countries for condemnation, nor to promote nationalistic hubris in which one country is seen as 'better', or 'more humane' than another. The issues affecting refugee children in our own times are cross national and the measures of control and treatment can be found in general terms across the industrialised world. The limitations identified in many programmes are not so much the products of weakness in national responses (although in some cases they are) as symptomatic of wider deficiencies that can be found across several countries. Likewise, no country is devoid of innovative and positive responses towards the care of refugee children and these are often achieved in the context of similar institutional and financial challenges.

The book as such is oriented primarily around particular themes rather than practices within specific countries and governed by overriding questions regarding the treatment of refugee children entering industrialised countries. I have adopted the term 'industrialised' following its common usage by international bodies such as UNHCR to encompass the countries of the European Union, North America, Australia and New Zealand. While there are references to a number of countries as illustrative of particular approaches to policy and practice, some have received considerably more extensive treatment than others. This is, as indicated above, partly due to a focus on themes rather than particular countries. It is also a consequence of selecting topics and locations of which I have the closest knowledge through various projects of collaborative research and educational exchange.

This knowledge has been generated through my experience in working on a wide variety of studies including an examination of good practice in mental health and social care of refugees in four European countries – UK, the Netherlands, Spain and Portugal – plus Australia, Canada and Guatemala (Watters *et al.*, 2003); an ongoing collaborative project on schools' projects for refugee children with colleagues at McGill University in Montreal and a review of policies of deterrence and their impact on refugees with colleagues at the University of New South Wales in Sydney (Silove *et al.*, 2000). It has also been influenced by engagement in a number of studies and educational forums with governmental bodies and NGOs including the Red Cross, the Refugee Council, various local authorities including Kent and Manchester, the Medical Foundation for the Care of Victims of Torture, the Transcultural Centre in Stockholm, the Nordic School of Public Health and the European Network of Asylum Reception Organisations.

Refugee children: issues of definition and enumeration

Academic and policy papers on refugees frequently begin with statements concerning the number of refugees in the world or, depending on the scope of the paper, in a specific geographical area. However, statistical presentations can be fraught with problems and data has to be carefully contextualised to avoid confusion. One salient distinction is between refugees and 'persons of concern' to the UNHCR. In 2003, for example, the global number of refugees reached an estimated 9.7 million while the total population of concern to UNHCR was 17.1 million. At the start of 2005, the figure for the number of people of concern had risen to 19.2 million, an increase of 13 per cent, while the number of refugees – identified as those who have fled persecution to seek safety by crossing international borders – had decreased by 4 per cent to 9.2 million people. Significant influences on the decline in refugee numbers in early 2005 included the return home of approximately one million Afghans and significant refugee returns to Iraq, Burundi, Angola and Liberia.

As noted above, persons 'of concern' include asylum seekers who may be defined as those who flee their own country and seek sanctuary in another state. Despite widespread concerns about an influx of large numbers of asylum seekers, the latter only constitutes about 4 per cent of the population of concern with the numbers of people seeking asylum in industrialised countries has declined significantly. In 2004 the number of asylum seekers, some 680,000, represented a fall to its lowest level for 16 years (UNHCR 2006a). The reasons behind this dramatic decrease in numbers are complex and contested. They are at least in part linked to the expansion of policies of deterrence, making it increasingly difficult for asylum seekers to cross international borders. For example, the UK, which in recent years has been a major country of destination, has taken a number of steps to deter asylum seekers, including tightening of borders, increasing visa restrictions in 'sending' countries, increasing fines for transport companies and restricting opportunities for pursuing asylum claims through the legal system. It is perhaps notable that France, often a major route for refugees heading towards the UK, displaced the UK in 2004 as the industrialised country receiving the highest number of asylum applications, some 58,500, as compared to a UK figure of 40,600.

An increasingly significant population 'of concern' to UNHCR is internally displaced people, commonly referred to as IDPs. Indeed at the present time, the ratio of IDPs to refugees is estimated to be 2.5:1 (Weiss and Korn, 2006, p12). UNHCR record that 'while nearly 5.6 million internally displaced persons were "of concern" to UNHCR in 2004, the total number of internally displaced persons worldwide was estimated at 25 million' (UNHCR, 2006b, p17). The circumstances of this group are likely to be similar to those of refugees with the exception that they have not crossed an international border in seeking safety from persecution. Columbia records the highest numbers of IDPs being helped by UNHCR, some 2 million according to government estimates and 3.3 million according to the estimates of NGOs. Other significant categories include stateless persons (approximately 2 million in 2004); some 1.5 million returnees who have gone back to countries of origin and a population of 83,700 in 2004 who have resettled, notably in Australia and the US.

Questions regarding the number and distribution of refugee children must be placed in this broader context. According to the UNHCR, in 2003 43 per cent of the population of concern of 17.1 million were under 18 years old. Eleven per cent were under the age of five. In Africa and the CASWANAME region (Central Asia, South-West Asia, North Africa and the Middle East) birth rates tend to be high and more than half of the refugee population is under 18 years old, with lower proportions in Asia and the Pacific (36%), Europe (26%) and the Americas (20%). These numbers fluctuate year on year and month by month, reflecting human responses to war, human rights violations and environmental catastrophes. It should be added that these figures include those IDPs helped by UNHCR, representing just over one fifth of the estimated 25 million IDPs worldwide (UNHCR, 2004).

A 2001 report by UNHCR entitled '*Women, Children and Older Refugees*' provides a relatively detailed and nuanced account of the global situation (UNHCR, 2001). The figures presented are broadly consistent with later reports in highlighting Africa as the region with the highest number of refugee children, with 17 per cent of the children under five and 56 per cent of the total global population of refugee children under 18. Here it is reported that the countries with the highest proportion of refugee children under five are Togo (26%) and Burundi (24%). However, aggregated data derived from continents may obscure salient differences between countries in the same region. For example, while 12 per cent of refugee children were located in Asia, high rates of refugee children under five were recorded in Bangladesh (24%) and East Timor (24%), similar to the rates in some African countries. In Europe, significant regional variations were noted in 2000, with children comprising almost half of the refugee population in Europe as a whole while representing only 21 per cent of the refugee population in Croatia and 17 per cent in the Federal Republic of Yugoslavia.

This disparity in numbers found between and within regions and countries, reflects broader contextual factors relating to refugee populations. They are based on numbers reported by UNHCR country offices and draw on various sources including 'governments, UNHCR and implementing partners' (UNHCR, 2001). UNHCR acknowledges that the reporting of numbers is uneven and 'in some cases, the data was collected under adverse conditions affecting the accuracy and reliability of the information' (UNHCR, 2001, p1). The significant differences in numbers of refugee children are not, however, simply a consequence of problems of data collection; they reflect responses to adversities arising in different regions in often dramatic and unpredictable ways. They also reflect the processes adopted by UNHCR and governments to identify populations as refugees or persons of concern and, by virtue of this designation, to be assisted by international and national programmes. There is, in short, a process whereby groups are identified as refugees with attendant processes of codification and classification. The extent of the presence of refugee children in any area thus reflects both the demographic characteristics of the groups in question and the mechanisms and scope of humanitarian missions.

These processes of classification and codification have been the subject of sustained attention from a number of scholars who stress the importance of subjecting statistical presentations to critical scrutiny. The social anthropologist Aiwa Ong, in a study of Cambodian refugees, draws on the work of Foucault to describe the mechanisms whereby refugees are identified as a distinctive population and objects of knowledge by governmental and non-governmental organisations. She refers to the aims and scope of her study in the following terms; 'What is at stake is the definition of the modern anthropos or human being by rational forms and techniques that converge in an identifiable problem-space' (Ong, 2003, p6). These 'rational forms and techniques' include the mechanisms for identifying and classifying refugees in camps and assessing levels of need in the pre- and post-migration contexts. In commenting on the situations of Vietnamese refugees in camps, John Knudsen similarly refers to the mechanisms whereby 'receiving countries rank individuals according to an elaborate system of classification' with resettlement opportunities implicitly influenced by considerations of class and education (Knudsen, 1995, p20). More broadly, systems of classification are predicated upon primary processes of enumeration under which predetermined categories of persons of concern form categories such as refugees, asylum seekers or IDPs.

Within this context UNHCR identifies as a distinctive category separated children defined as 'children under 18 years of age who are separated from both parents or from their previous legal or customary primary caregiver' (UNHCR, 2004). As noted above, refugee children may be seen as representing a distinct group within a broader category of displaced children. Strictly speaking, becoming a refugee child depends on a process of according a specific legal status to a child who has crossed an international border and is deemed individually, or as part of a family, as having a well-founded fear of persecution. Being a refugee child is thus an *ascribed* identity temporally defined as relating normally to the ages of 0–17 years based on Western conceptions of childhood and the transition to adulthood. As such it is based on universalised notions of the child and the span of childhood, which may be quite different to those operating in the countries of origin of refugee children. While socially and culturally constructed, the categorising of a refugee as a child may have wide ranging resonance in terms of asylum procedures, education and welfare support and approaches to social integration. The refugee in his or her late teens may thus, possibly unwittingly, stand at a critical junction in which processes of age determination may have a crucial impact on their lives.

More specifically, being viewed as a child as opposed to a refugee adult, may result in a range of different specialists or specialist bodies having primary responsibility for areas of health, education and welfare support. In the case of unaccompanied asylum-seeking children and refugees, distinct agencies may be responsible for welfare and housing. A further implication is that, in the area of social care, care giving will be underpinned by theories of child development developed over decades in the West.

In the following chapters, the responses of immigration authorities and services towards refugee children are examined. An early focus is on children within border areas, drawing particularly on examples from southern Europe. The analysis then follows and, to some degree, parallels the journeys taken by refugee children to northern Europe and the UK. Specific locations are investigated to explore broader themes in social care responses to refugee children that are more broadly illustrative of situations in a number of countries. The ports of Calais, Zeebrugge and Dover illustrate the various responses of immigration and social care agencies in deterring or incorporating refugee children. These include mechanisms of what I refer to as non-incorporation, whereby children are deterred from making asylum claims, to various ways in which children are incorporated through programmes aimed at social and emotional well-being and dispersal.

Following the investigation of children at borders, attention is given to the area of 'social care' broadly conceptualised to encompass arrangements pertaining to dispersal and accommodation, health care and education. A number of distinctive discourses are identified that are highly influential in locating children within what Ong has referred to as 'problem-spaces' (2003, p6) and organising their care. These discourses are reflected in the development of a range of international programmes that are designed to address refugee children's psychosocial and emotional problems. One influential group of programmes offered by Pharos in the Netherlands provides a basis for the examination of this distinctive type of response to refugee children. The later chapters of the book offer a wider analysis of features of good practice in the social care of refugee children as well as offering a synthesis of salient theoretical approaches. The book concludes with the presentation of seven accomplishments that attempt to consolidate the emerging findings into a practical programme of action in the field. Before embarking on an examination of the treatment of refugee children at borders, an overview of relevant theoretical aspects is presented.

2 Theoretical orientations

Migration and refugee children

Migration is a wide-ranging, multifaceted and highly complex phenomenon and is appropriately approached through interdisciplinary research. Brettell and Hollifield have identified a range of disciplinary approaches to the subject highlighting the importance of contributions from sociology, anthropology, demography, political science and economics (Brettell and Hollifield, 2000). Much research in the field by political scientists focuses on the questions relating to the causes and scale of migration. In a highly influential paper, the political theorist Aristide Zolberg has highlighted the influence of national policies aimed at restricting the flow of migrants as having a decisive influence on patterns of migration in the modern era (Zolberg, 1989). As such, he shifted focus from neo-classical theories, such as those proposed by Ravenstein, which emphasised movements as influenced by factors such as population density and economic opportunities. Drawing on a wide range of disciplinary perspectives, Stephen Castles and Mark Miller in their influential book, *The Age of Migration*, have presented four theoretical and methodological orientations with respect to migration; push/pull theories, historical/structuralist theories, migration systems theories, and transnational theory (Castles and Miller, 2003). It is useful to outline these here and consider their potential contribution to research on refugee children.

While presented by Castles and Miller under the broad category of economic theories of migration, what are commonly presented as push/pull theories are influential in a range of disciplines including demography and sociology. Push/pull theories conceptualise migration as the product of two interrelated processes. Push factors are those that decisively influence a decision to leave one's homeland. These may include poor economic or educational prospects, high population density, environmental catastrophe (e.g. flooding, severe environmental degradation making it impossible to sustain traditional lifestyles) or persecution by state or non-state agencies. Pull factors may include perception of good economic opportunities, the presence of family or community members in the proposed country of migration, language, a sense of the country of migration as safe and secure. Push/pull theories are influenced by neo-classical economic theory and are underpinned by a notion of the migrant as a rational agent weighing up the pros and cons of the situation in his or her home country and of the country of migration. According to Castles and Miller, 'Its central concept is "human capital": people decide to invest in migration, in the same way as they might invest in education or vocational training, because it raises their human capital and brings potential future gains in earnings' (2003, p23). While push/pull theories have proved useful in analysing various forms of migration, they do have some weaknesses when considering forced migration. They fail to take account of the circumstances of forced migration in which migrants may have little or no choice either about leaving their home country or concerning the country of migration. They also often do not address the reasons why migrants who do have choice settle in particular countries that are densely populated or where there are not significant economic advantages.

The second approach identified by Castles and Miller is 'historical-structural', which they describe as informed by Marxist political economy, and stresses the unequal economic and political power in the world economy. It uses the presence of gross economic inequalities between 'developed' and 'developing' countries as a basis for explaining migratory flows. The approach has some obvious strengths, for example, in providing an explanatory model for understanding the movement of migrant mine workers to South Africa, or the movement of Turks to Germany as 'guest workers'. However, while in broad terms, one could argue that many migratory flows are ultimately determined by macro economic factors, this approach alone is unlikely to provide an adequate explanation for specific flows; why particular groups migrate to particular countries. As such, it does not engage with factors that could help to explain why, for example, a Kurdish family may have migrated to the UK, rather than to Germany or France.

An attempt to offer a more comprehensive approach is represented by 'migration systems theory' which seeks to integrate macro-level factors involving the relationship between countries and economies and micro-level factors that attempt to pay appropriate attention to the migrants themselves and their decision-making processes. This approach recognises migration as a consequence of interrelated macro and micro factors and stresses the importance of an integrated and interdisciplinary focus. According to Castles and Miller:

> The basic principle is that any migratory movement can be seen as a result of interacting macro and micro structures. Macro-structures refer to large-scale institutional factors, while micro-structures embrace the networks, practices and beliefs of the migrants themselves. These two levels are linked by a number of intermediate mechanisms, which are often referred to as meso-structures.
>
> (Castles and Miller, 2003, p27)

These structures interrelate within a migration system which includes 'two or more countries which exchange migrants with each other' (ibid., p26). This suggests an enduring relationship that, on many occasions, includes periods of colonial rule. Thus, the presence of Surinamese in the Netherlands is related to colonial history, as is the presence of Indians, Pakistanis and Bangladeshis in the UK and the presence of Algerians in France. The micro structures here also suggest a durable temporal dimension, manifested through the formation of kinship and social networks that extend between the countries. This durability is supported by the presence of meso-level actors, who in Castles and Miller's exposition constitute something of a 'migration industry' and includes 'recruitment organisations, lawyers, agents, smugglers and other intermediaries'. The presence of this industry has 'often confounded government efforts to control or stop movements' (ibid.). Moreover, migration systems theory suggests a research agenda oriented towards multi-level and interdisciplinary approaches that explore the interrelationship between macro, meso and micro structures.

Interdisciplinary approaches are also suggested by the fourth theoretical approach, transnational theory. This body of research addresses the phenomenon of 'circulatory or repeated mobility, in which people migrate regularly between a number of places where they have economic, social or cultural linkages' (ibid., p29). It also examines the maintenance of national identity in deterritorialised contexts, through the utilisation of new technologies of communication. Lucy Williams' recent research has, for example, examined the part played by mobile phones and the Internet among Kurdish and Afghan refugees in England. Despite being unable to be in the physical presence of Kurdish and Afghan friends and family, nevertheless a sense of community identity was maintained and assumed increasing significance around major life events such as marriages, births and deaths (Williams, 2006). The anthropologist Arjun Appadurai has made significant contributions to the debate on deterritorialisation, stressing both its economic determinants and its political impacts on the country of migration and the country of origin. 'Deterritorialization', he argues,

> in general, is one of the central forces of the modern world because it brings labouring populations into the lower-class sectors and spaces of relatively wealthy societies, while sometimes creating exaggerated and intensified senses of criticism or attachment to politics in the home state.
>
> (Appadurai, 1996, p37)

A further example of a transnational approach is concerned particularly with the field of social care. Elaine Bauer and Paul Thompson have examined the development of Jamaican Mutual Aid. Drawing on extensive fieldwork in both Jamaica and the UK, Bauer and Thompson examine the way in which family roles have developed and are maintained in transnational contexts and challenge prevailing stereotypes that view migration as a one-way process from the developing to the developed world. Care of the elderly and of children is, for example, often realised in transcultural contexts. Commenting on the latter, they observe that,

> help with children...operates in almost all our families, and in over half of them there are transnational instances. Sometimes it is a response to a disaster, such as parental death; but more often it is a positive strategy chosen so as to

help the young adult parent get into work, or to get ahead as a migrant. Some children are also sent back to kin in Jamaica in the hope of a better education.

They observe that,

> While the key axis of exchanges of help is between parents, children and grandchildren, it is notable how the possibilities extend well beyond this. Aunts are common care givers. Cousins are taken in to assist migrants. Remittances are sent not only to parents, but often also to siblings or to in-laws. Temporary help with migration may extend to very distant kin, including even ex-in-laws.
>
> (Bauer and Thompson, 2006, p45)

While Appadurai highlights the way in which ethnic and national identities endure and may indeed be both strengthened and transformed in a deterritorialised context, Bauer and Thompson emphasise the impact of family ties and the specific ways in which these are animated in support of migrants. As such, they provide a specific example of transnational aspects in the functioning of social support and social care, areas normally considered within circumscribed geographical localities.

The theoretical approaches outlined by Castles and Miller are addressed towards an understanding of migration as a whole and it is useful to consider the extent to which they illuminate the particular situations of refugee children. Push/pull theories are, as noted above, characterised as linked to rational choice and an immediate response would be that they are of limited use in understanding situations where parents or other adult relatives are likely to make decisions about migration in contexts in which children are fleeing from a country. However, in some forced migration contexts, they may help illuminate the decision making of adults, particularly where decisions are made to send children to another country. Unaccompanied asylum-seeking children arrive in a number of industrialised countries having often had their trips paid for by adult relatives hoping to give them a safe environment and a better opportunity in life. The process of sending the child may be viewed as rational in that it may have included an estimation of his or her life chances in the home country, an assessment of the options for trans- port to another country and an assessment of the most desirable country for the child. As discussed in Chapter 3, Derluyn and Broekaert from the University of Ghent have observed on the basis of fieldwork in the port of Zeebrugge in Belgium, the unaccompanied minors passing through the port often have a very clear objective – to get to the UK. It is seen as the 'promised land' and this has been an objective that has been present since the initial stages of their journey (Derluyn and Broekaert, 2005).

It is probably fair to assess push/pull theories as helpful in some instances and less so in others. For example, the situation of a child sent by relatively wealthy parents from Afghanistan to Europe to seek a safer and more promising life may be usefully analysed in this way. However, it is a less useful approach in considering the case of people who have fled from immediate and ongoing violent persecution, where there may not have been many, if any, alternative courses of action. A process of rational choice suggests the availability of human capital and this may be sorely lacking in many of the emergency situations refugees face (Van Hear, 2006).

A historical-structural approach is, as noted above, addressed towards understanding the global political and economic forces that drive migration. As such, it offers a useful perspective on the factors giving rise to child refugees. The way in which economic and social inequalities are created and sustained through world economic systems form an important backdrop to understanding the forces that lead to forced migration. The sociologist Zygmunt Bauman presents a compelling account of the interrelationships between economic progress and globalisation and the emergence of economic migrants, asylum seekers and refugees. The economic systems of modernity, he argues, have created surplus and outcast populations who, deprived of opportunities in their own countries, desperately seek opportunities elsewhere. Bauman characterises this 'surplus population' as the 'unintended and unplanned 'collateral casualties' of economic progress.

> In the course of economic progress...the extant forms of 'making a living' are successively dismantled, broken up into components meant to be reassembled ('recycled') into new forms. In the process some components are damaged beyond repair, while of those that survive the dismantling phase, only a reduced quantity is needed to compose the new, as a rule smarter and slimmer, working contraptions.
>
> (Bauman, 2004, p39)

Here asylum seekers and economic migrants are presented as produced directly, albeit unwittingly, by the mechanisms of modern global capitalism.

A similar perspective is offered by Manual Castells, in the context of his highly influential studies of the 'Information Age'. In *End of Millennium*, the third volume of his well-known trilogy, Castells identifies what he views as remarkable and distinctive features of the last quarter of the twentieth century,

> A dynamic, global economy has been constituted around the planet, linking up valuable people and activities from all over the world, while switching off from the networks of power and wealth, people and territories dubbed as irrelevant from the perspective of dominant interests.
>
> (Castells, 2000, p1)

The latter he identifies as constituting a 'Fourth World', which, while located in many of the poorest countries on the planet, is not geographically determined.

> The Fourth World comprises large areas of the globe, such as much of sub-Saharan Africa, and impoverished rural areas of Latin America and Asia. But it is also present in literally every country, and every city, in this new geography of social exclusion. It is formed of American inner-city ghettos, Spanish enclaves of mass youth unemployment, French banlieues warehousing North Africans, Japanese Yoseba quarters, and Asian mega-cities' shanty towns.
>
> (Castells, 2000, p168)

Castells' deterritorialising of the social spaces of poverty and marginalisation challenges ubiquitous views of the world's social and economic problems as located principally in 'Third World' countries, and draws attention to the poverty of both migrant and autochthonous populations in parts of the 'developed world'.

Castells employs similar language to Baumann in referring to the situation of children inhabiting this 'Fourth World' at the end of the twenty-first century. They are viewed here as 'wasted' as a consequence of the 'unchecked characteristics of informational capitalism'. What we are witnessing, according to him, is a 'dramatic reversal of social conquests and children's rights obtained by social reform in mature industrial societies in the wake of large scale deregulation and the bypassing of governments by global networks' (ibid., p162). In contrast to the push/pull dichotomy proposed by some migration theorists, Castells depicts children as caught between 'supply and demand' factors. On the one hand there is supply of children brought about by a breakdown of family structures, poverty and misery resulting in children being 'sold for survival, are sent to the streets to help out, or end up running away from the hell of their homes to the hell of their non-existence' (ibid., p163). Demand is created by the processes of globalisation, business networking, criminalisation of a segment of the economy, and advanced communication technologies. A further crucially interrelated factor in children's exploitation and exclusion is the 'disintegration of states and societies, and the massive uprooting of populations by war, famine, epidemics, and banditry' (ibid., p164).

While Castells offers a substantial and compelling analysis of the position of children at the beginning of the new millennium, there is an overriding tendency to see children of the Fourth World solely in the context of victims of powerful socio-economic forces existing, in his words, in the 'black holes of informational capitalism'. There is, of course, a considerable degree of truth in his analysis and it would be both naïve and trivialising to suggest that an overriding emphasis should be placed on children's agency in the context of situations of extreme poverty and destitution. It is vitally important that writers of the calibre of Castells identify the pernicious effects of globalisation and contemporary capitalism on potentially vulnerable groups, including children. However, the picture presented here is incomplete in a number of ways. For example, the image of government as the potential protector of children being swept aside by the forces of the new capitalism does not take into account the potential impact of 'meso-' level actors. National governments are frequently held to account and exhorted to improve the well-being of children by international bodies armed with standards of good practice. Moreover, as a range of studies has shown, even in the most extreme circumstances, children adopt strategies to interpret and cope with the realities around them. To take but one of a number of possible examples, Eyber and Ager conclude on the basis of their research of young people's experiences of the war in Angola that

> the youths in this study were astute analysts of their situation and had insight into the interrelatedness of factors...approaches that view children predominantly as passive recipients of aid and care frequently do not

recognise this ability of the young to contribute valuable perspectives on the dimensions of war.

(Eyber and Ager, 2004, p205)

Boyden and de Berry on the basis of their studies of children in conflict zones, argue that 'children and adolescents can be very active in defining their own allegiances during conflict, as well as their own strategies for coping and survival (Boyden and de Berry 2004, p15).

In summary, while Castells and Bauman offer compelling insights into the effects of contemporary capitalism, there is a tendency in some of their writings to present migrants, both economic and refugees, solely in the circumscribed role of victims of globalisation.[1] As such, their analysis reflects some weaknesses in the historical-structural approach outlined above. In this particular context, there is little sense of the role of human agency, of the way in which refugees make sense of their world and act upon it. As a number of studies referred to above have shown, whilst external political and economic circumstances may define the environment in which refugee children are placed, they are simultaneously meaningful interpreters of that environment. The historical-structuralist orientation involves little engagement with what Richard Sennett refers to as 'taking people seriously as competent interpreters of their own lives', learning how 'subjects make sense of themselves' (Sennett, 2006, p4).

As noted above, what Castles and Miller refer to as 'migration systems theory' offers the potential of bridging the gap between macro analysis of social and political factors and a micro level in which migrants and refugees make decisions about leaving their homelands and seeking protection elsewhere. By focusing on the interrelationships between particular countries as components of a 'system' in which migration takes place, there are opportunities for examining in depth the interplay of salient historical, economic, cultural and social factors at both the macro and micro levels. To develop an understanding of the example of, say, an Afghan adolescent boy who arrives as an asylum seeker in the UK in 2006, one may appropriately take into consideration macro-level factors such as the historical involvement of Britain and other Western powers in Afghanistan culminating in the military action against the Taliban in 2001. The boy's flight would be seen in the broader context of continuing instability in Afghanistan and serious ongoing deficiencies in the provision of education, health care and social welfare. However, an understanding of the boy's situation also requires an examination of micro-level factors, including the reasons why he has come to the UK. Is this where he had planned to come? Who had financed and supported him to undertake the trip? Does he have relatives and friends in the UK?

One can see that migration systems theory offers, in broad terms, a useful theoretical framework for the analysis of refugee children's concrete situations. It does have some potential deficiencies, however. In focusing on the interrelationships between specific countries with close historical ties, it may do little to illuminate the broader global aspects of migration. To return to the above example, the conflict in Afghanistan commencing in 2001, while broadly related to the entanglement of

European powers in the history of the country, is more clearly related to American-led action against the Taliban and Al-Qaeda in the wake of the attack on the World Trade Center buildings in New York. Longer-term historical ties between the countries may have resulted in the presence of a relatively small Afghani community in the UK with whom the boy has some affinity and which could offer some support. However, arguably the strongest explanations for the boy's flight to the UK lie in recent events and circumstances rather than historically durable ties between these specific countries.

Transnational theories relate, as noted above, to the maintenance of ties and communities in deterritoralised contexts. They provide powerful perspectives on the ways in which bonds of nationhood and community are maintained in a globalised world. In the context of research on refugee children, they highlight ways in which cultural norms and practices can be maintained, despite an absence of physical proximity to communities. However, the emphasis in this approach is on the maintenance of bonds and networks rather than their dissolution, and there is a danger that an overriding concern with demonstrating the ways in which communities are maintained ignores vital processes linked to the erosion of traditional bonds and the development of new networks.

Something of this erosion is witnessed by the anthropologist Lisa Malkki, in her influential study of Hutu refugees in Tanzania. Here she demonstrates that some refugees, instead of surviving in camps, move to urban areas in which they try to forget past ties and the memory of persecution. Malkki argues that the town refugees' relationship to their 'mythico-history' was not so much one of denial as an 'indefinite suspension of history'. Moreover, for the town refugees, the past 'had simply passed, it was not a predominating, structuring force in their everyday lives in a positive sense...' as it was for the refugees in camps (Malkki, 1995, p194). Within transnational theories overriding concerns with investigating the ways in which traditions and allegiances are maintained may also obscure the circumstances of individual refugees. Some have fled owing to holding minority or marginal views and orientations that may make them ill-disposed towards maintaining links with the majority of countrymen and women, and perhaps even their ethnic group, clan or family members. Religious affiliation or conversion may, for example, have alienated a family from their community, or an individual may have been isolated and endangered owing to his or her sexual orientation.

In conclusion, the four theoretical models put forward by Castles and Miller all have some potential strengths in terms of analysing the movements of refugee children. The phenomenon in question is varied and complex and efforts to encapsulate it within any single theoretical framework risk ignoring some important factors. Migration systems theory has the merit of viewing migration in terms of an interrelationship between macro and micro factors and this provides a useful orientation for addressing the complexities involved in the movement of refugee children. An engagement with theories of migration orientates us towards an understanding of the motivations and pressures on children to migrate. However, an examination of the ways in which they are treated by institutions and services requires further theoretical considerations.

Theorising refugee childhoods

James and colleagues have pointed out that sociological interest in childhood itself is a relatively recent phenomenon, with interest previously largely subsumed under other topics such as the family or schooling (James *et al.*, 1998, p22). One particularly influential theoretical orientation in recent decades has been the examination of the socially constructed child. According James *et al.*, to describe childhood as socially constructed is to 'suspend a belief in, or a willing reception of, its taken-for-granted meanings' (1998, p26). A social constructivist approach involves scrutiny of accepted norms and predispositions and of the way in which these have developed in specific social, political, historical and moral contexts. Social constructivists' purpose is to 'go back to the phenomenon in consciousness and show how it is built up. So, within a social constructive, idealist world there are no essential forms or constraints' (James *et al.*, 1998 p26). As such, it represents an approach that contrasts with what James and James have termed the 'social-structural child', a conception of the child and childhood that is underpinned by both the formal institutions of the law but also, as invoked through a more capacious concept of what the authors term 'Law', 'the less formal processes and mechanisms that exist in all societies, both religious and secular' (James and James, 2004, p49). A social constructivist perspective necessarily involves the study of these processes including the way in which concepts of the child and childhood are formulated and enshrined in social and political discourses. Social practice routinely, and arguably necessarily, 'deals with childhood as a universal but specific social and legal category which is, and needs to be, distinguishable from adulthood' (ibid., p65).

The ubiquity of the social constructivist approach has been noted by the sociologist Nikolas Rose who observed that it is now commonplace to describe the objects of science as socially constructed. However, he argues that the language of social construction is often weak. Drawing on Foucault, suggests that the interesting question is not whether objects are socially constructed, but how they are constructed. 'Where do objects emerge? Which are the authorities who are able to pronounce upon them? Through what concepts and explanatory regimes are they specified? How do certain constructions acquire the status of truth...?' (Rose, 1999a, pp10–11). Indeed a further, and increasingly prominent, range of studies in the migration field is influenced by the work of Foucault. These include the studies of Malkki, referred to above, but also recent work by Ong (2003), Fassin (2001), Morris (1998) and Inda (2006) among others. Foucault's work is extensive and particular aspects of it have proven influential to those studying forced and irregular migration. In particular these commonly draw on Foucault's work on governmentality and subjectivity. Foucault describes the former as:

> The ensemble formed by the institutions, procedures, analysis and reflections, the calculations and tactics that allow the exercise of this very specific

albeit complex form of power, which has as its target population, as its principle form of knowledge political economy, and as its essential technical
means apparatuses of security.

(Foucault, 1991, p102)

In Ong's study of Cambodian refugees in the US, she describes Foucault as arguing that 'advanced liberal societies tend to depend on regulation rather than
discipline; they rely on human-science policy and techniques to "govern through
freedom", thereby inducing citizen-subjects to become self-motivated, self-
reliant, and entrepreneurial' (Ong, 2003, p7). She thus elaborates on the important
link Foucault makes between the apparatus of governments and the emergence of
personal dispositions and subjectivities. It may be useful, without being too formulaic, to paraphrase Foucault and characterise governmentality as consisting of
three vitally interrelated components: the apparatus of government (laws, policies
and procedures etc.), the human sciences or 'complex of savoirs' that support
government, and the dispositions and behaviours of the population, specifically
the ways in which it becomes 'self-governing'. An orientation towards these areas
of investigation has underpinned a number of useful studies in the field.

The work of Ong (2003) has applied a governmentality perspective to both pre-
and post-migration contexts not only by examining the ways in which refugees were
screened in camps on the Thai border to determine who were the 'good refugees',
but also how the processes initiated in the camps represented an initial attempt to
introduce American norms and values to the Cambodians. A substantial part of
Ong's study concerns the post-migration environment, particularly the interface
between the refugees and US social and health services. Her analytical framework
incorporates an approach to the conceptualisation and examination of citizenship
that is distinctly Foucauldian. Her aim is to examine the 'technologies of government – that is the policies, programs, codes and practices...that attempt to instil in
citizen-subjects particular values (self-reliance, freedom, individualism, calculation
or flexibility) in a variety of domains' (Ong, 2003, p276). Ong's concern, however,
is not only with the pervasiveness of technologies of government, but also with the
strategies people adopt in responding to these technologies. She describes, for
example, how 'women's newfound voices – stories that fitted controlling narratives
about being a refugee, welfare recipient, or victim of domestic violence – did not
preclude efforts on their part to deflect and question American values'. Similarly
refugee children were far from passive recipients of American norms and values,
they 'learned to navigate the rules and play off different sources of authority (patri-
archal, psychiatric, legal) in pursuit of their own interests' (Ong, 2003, p279).

Lisa Malkki's influential work on refugees, like Ong's, draws significantly on
the work of Foucault and pursues an 'archaeology of knowledge' to examine the
way in which the category of the refugee is discursively produced. Malkki's influential book, *Purity and Exile*, referred to above, draws on extensive fieldwork
among Hutu refugees in Tanzania. She argues that Foucauldian methods are particularly productive in the study of refugees.

Just as Foucault has shown for prisons and clinics, the refugee camp as a technology of power was both limiting and productive. Within it, certain kinds of political action were possible, others impossible. Certain kinds of socio-political forms and processes, and certain kinds of objects and subjects, emerged while others did not

(Malkki, 1995, p237)

Beyond the refugee camp, Malkki has commented more widely on the emergence of the refugee as an 'epistemic object in construction'. She suggests that it would be inappropriate to search back to earlier epochs in an attempt to trace the origins of the refugee as an ideal type or, in her words, a 'proto-refugee'. Rather,

there is no 'proto-refugee' of which the modern refugee is a direct descendent, any more than there is a proto-nation of which the contemporary nation form is a logical, inevitable outgrowth. Instead of constructing such false continuities we might do better to locate historical moments of reconfiguration at which whole new objects can appear.

(Malkki, 1995b, p497)

She argues that, while people have always sought refuge and sanctuary, in terms of modern formulations, the refugee emerged after World War Two. It was then that 'a more encompassing apparatus of administrative procedures' emerged beyond circumscribed treaties and protocols for dealing with specific displaced populations.

Malkki's historicism underpins broader theoretical and methodological concerns regarding the nature and scope of refugee studies. Her extensive review of the field suggests that studies of refugees may share the following interrelated characteristics: the presentation of the 'refugee experience' as though it was homogenous and consisting of distinctive identifiable stages; the routine incorporation of the language of loss (e.g. of traditions, culture, identity) as a consequence of becoming a refugee; the prominence of psychological interpretations of displacement. Against these prevailing tendencies, she argues for a more nuanced, reflexive and, arguably, politically engaged approach. Invoking Foucault's exhortations towards an engaged and critical international citizenship, she argues for a 'denaturalising, questioning stance towards the national order of things' that includes questioning the sense of emplacement as well as displacement and related questions of nationality, citizenship and the sovereign state (ibid., p517). This implies a theoretical and methodological orientation towards research that does not begin from relatively uncritical presuppositions regarding the nature of refugees or the refugee experience, but from an examination of a broader picture in which the category 'refugee' emerges as an object of knowledge and of practice.

Given the importance of Malkki's contribution to the field, it is appropriate to examine the implications of this approach in a little more detail and, specifically, the implications for research on refugee children. Firstly, of course, it implies that the category 'refugee children' is not taken as an uncritical basis for research. One should examine the contexts in which the category emerges and the apparatuses of administrative procedures within which it operates. It is useful analytically to distinguish different governmental and bureaucratic 'levels' in which the category emerges, from transnational institutions such as the UN, to national governments, local government and non-governmental organisations. Salient questions here include examination of the circumstances in which governmental and non-governmental organisations distinguish refugee children as a distinctive group and the way in which their needs are perceived. It is also important to examine policies and practices aimed at refugee children through questions such as How are they constituted? Which public bodies are held responsible for refugee children's welfare? What shape does this welfare provision take? How do discourses of assimilation and integration inform practices?

Besides the role of government, a range of professional specialists formulate theories, offer advice and deliver services to refugee children. These include professionals working in refugee camps, reception centres and community resources in host societies incorporating, for example, teachers, educationalists, psychologists, doctors, nurses and social workers. Besides the policies and practices of the organisations for which they work, they are expected to comply with the professional standards associated with their positions and enshrined in a variety of codes of practice. Their professional bodies may, in addition to having guidelines for working with children, have specific procedures that relate to refugee children and which are informed by distinctive perceptions of their needs. They may also have specific policies and guidelines in relation to minority ethnic groups according to which practices towards refugee children should comply. It is important here to reiterate that refugee children as distinguished in a legal sense constitute a distinctive group whose rights and opportunities are likely to be considerably enhanced when compared to those of asylum seekers or irregular migrants. An approach consistent with that advocated by Malkki would include the contexts and manner in which these groups are distinguished and the attendant implications for their social care.

While critics have acknowledged the value of Foucauldian approaches to the analysis of power, his approach has been criticised for giving little attention to the ways in which people may respond to forms of oppression. The political scientist Seyla Benhabib in her book *The Claims of Culture*, characterises Foucault's approach as maintaining that 'all justificatory strategies, all pretences to philosophical objectivity are trapped within historical horizons and in cultural, social and psychological currents' (Benhabib, 2002, p26). Edward Said has pointed to limitations of Foucault's approach in describing him as a 'scribe of power' (Said, 2001) and, while admiring his method, felt Foucault had virtually given up on political struggle. Eagleton has criticised Foucault's approach along similar lines as 'exemplary of an ideology now dominant among a certain sector of the Western radical intelligentsia: libertarian pessimism' (Eagleton, 1990, p387).

However, as in Ong's work, Malkki identifies sites of *resistance* within the context of a Foucauldian analysis of power. She cites refugee camps alongside 'prisons, old-age institutions, mining compounds', as 'transformative technologies of power in which collectivities of persons become fixed and objectified as the "inmates", "the elderly", "the labour force", and "the refugees"'. She identifies the potential for resistance within these constraining environments, arguing that it is 'also relevant that such technologies of power can, and often do, become generative, productive sites for social and political intervention and transformation...' (Malkki, 1995a, p238). In stressing the active role of refugees themselves in interpreting and responding strategically to processes of governmentality, these scholars implicitly reject these criticisms and suggest that a Foucauldian approach does not necessarily preclude the potential for resistance.

In considering the specific practices directed towards refugee children by a range of welfare organisations including those concerned with health, accommodation and housing, it is helpful to consider these within the context of a moral economy of care. I previously evoked the concept of the moral economy to refer to the parameters within which the presence of asylum seekers was legitimated by governments and underpinned policies of dispersal (Watters, 2001b). Legitimation in this context reflects Thompson's definition in which it is linked to a belief in the defence of traditional rights and customs and supported by the wider consensus of the community (Thompson, 1971, p78). While the concept of the moral economy is often evoked in relation to pre-capitalist relations within traditional embedded economies within which there are strong relations of reciprocity (e.g. Booth 1994), here the concept is used in a slightly different way. Within the present context a moral economy may be seen as linked to the representation of asylum-seeker refugees as lacking in legitimacy in making demands on welfare provision. The moral economy is thus infused with beliefs that far from being victims of persecution, those who are making claims for support are manipulative and unscrupulous and as such lacking in a moral claim for economic support. This perspective may be seen as underpinning strategies of non incorporation and biolegitimacy that are explored in the ensuing chapters.

Cultural diversity and child development

Contemporary theories of child development are generally viewed as heavily influenced by the philosophical works of Rousseau and Locke. Locke argued that at birth a child is like a *tabula rasa* – a blank slate – subsequently written on by her or his experience. By contrast, Rousseau viewed children as possessed by innate characteristics such as a sense of right and wrong and having the ability to reason and make moral decisions. Orientations towards a view of children as influenced primarily by nature or nurture continue to underpin contemporary debate with emphasis on the one hand on the determining influence of genetics and, on the other, the influence of experience and education (Stainton Rogers, 2001, p203). While, as Rose has contended, the mind and behaviour of the growing child had been an object for psychological discussion prior to the 1920s, it was in this decade that 'the child became a scientific object for psychology by means of the concept of development' (Rose, 1998, p110). He describes the approach as follows:

The gathering of data on children of particular ages over a certain span, and the organising of these data into age norms, enabled the norms to be arranged along an axis of time, and seen as cross sections through a continuous dimension of development.

(Ibid., p110)

The scientific enterprise was crucially influenced by the institutional development of the clinic and the nursery. The process was highly normative and provided yardsticks for identifying aberrations and deviance as well as prescribing remedial action.

A potential deficiency in developmental approaches rests in their universalising of Western norms and values and imposing developmental trajectories by which children from all cultures are judged. An adherence, for example, to Bowlby's attachment theory presupposes a critical linkage between infant and mother without which the child faces deprivation and becomes frozen and withdrawn. The importance of attachment and the deleterious effects of separation were emphasised by Anna Freud and Dorothy Burlingham in their study of wartime child evacuees in the UK (1943). According to their findings, separation from mothers was more traumatising than the impact of exposure to air raids and bombings. While Freud and Burlingham provide compelling evidence to support their findings, a central concern in the present context is not whether their evidence is persuasive, but whether it is applicable cross-culturally. The finding that British children during the war were profoundly affected by separation from their mothers is derived from a specific historical and cultural context in which mothers had the predominant, and frequently sole, responsibility for childcare.

To generalise from such findings is ethnocentric, not least in failing to take account of the diversity of child-rearing practices in which the mother may not be the sole primary care giver. Studies in different cultural contexts have challenged the notion that the mother and child relationship always follows this pattern with, for example, findings from India demonstrating that children may have a number of relatives who assume a mothering role within the extended Hindu family (Kurtz, 1994). As early as 1928 Margaret Mead in her seminal and controversial work *Coming of Age in Samoa* had challenged the ubiquity and normative value of Western notions of child development (Mead, 2001). Recently Gillian Mann has pointed out that, while implicit notions of the mother as the primary caregiver are true in certain contexts, 'in many societies childcare is a social enterprise in which children have multiple caretakers and experience exclusive maternal care only in the first few months of life' (Mann, 2004, p10). The substantial impact of cultural factors is not reflected adequately in much of the research in that culture is examined only as an independent variable that may affect child development but not 'a system of meanings that creates alternative pathways for social, emotional and cognitive development' (ibid., p11).

Besides evidence of the diversity of culturally embedded norms and practices surrounding childhood and adolescents, historical research has demonstrated how concepts of the child and childhood have developed and changed over time. The historian Philippe Aries has located the origins of childhood in Europe in the mid-eighteenth century. According to James *et al.*'s exegesis, at this time

> adults in particular social classes were steadily beginning to think of themselves as of not quite the same order of being as their children. An age based hierarchy and eventual dichotomy was becoming institutionalised in the relationship between adults and children and the defining characteristics of these differences were, by and large, oppositional.
>
> (James *et al.*, 1998, p4)

Citing Richard Sennett, James *et al.* describe Aries' work as paving the way for 'the study of the family as a historical form, rather than as a fixed biological form in history' (ibid., p4).

Views of childhood as historically, socially and culturally contingent obviously raise questions regarding the appropriateness of employing models generated in specific Western social and cultural milieus to populations of refugee children from across the globe. The specificity of the Western approach to childhood is addressed provocatively by Scheper-Hughes and Sargent who argue that in contrast to what they refer to as the 'cherished myth of child centeredness in modern, industrialised, democratic societies', 'images of the child as an economic liability and a burden proliferate in the popular culture' (1998, p10). These are set in stark contrast to what the authors refer to as the 'child-saving and child rights discourses' that are exported by industrialised countries and welfare organisations. The authors challenge the prevailing orthodoxy that sees children in Western countries as inherently privileged by their access to consumer goods and education and avoidance of wage-labour. According to them: 'Children, now seen as family consumers rather than helpful proto-workers or apprentices...have been relegated to the status of family welfare recipients, resented and pitied as much as they are valued and protected' (ibid., p11).

The placing of discourses of childhood prevalent in industrialised countries in historical, cultural and socio-economic contexts encourages critical reflexivity with respect to practices directed towards refugee children. For example, the presupposed ubiquity of notions of time underpinning the developmental trajectory is far from universal. James *et al.* have pointed to the historical evolution of our notions of time and their interrelationship with the waning of agricultural modes of production and the advent of industrialisation. Indeed contemporary notions of time, evolved in late modernity, are subsequently challenging industrialised concepts of the working day and divisions between work and leisure time. In this context for example, research has highlighted the painful transition workers in industry face in developing more flexible working routines as a consequence of globalisation and the decline of traditional industries (Walkerdine, 2006).

Pierre Bourdieu in his seminal studies of agriculturally based societies in North Africa has analysed the interrelationship between agricultural production, the apprehension of temporal rhythms and the stages of life. Here he identified a 'social structuring of temporality' that fulfils a political function by symbolically manipulating *age limits* i.e. the boundaries that define age-groups, but also the limitations imposed on different ages. The mythico-ritual categories cut up the age continuum into discontinuous segments, constituted not biologically (like the physical signs of aging) but socially, and marked by the symbolism of cosmetics and clothing, decorations, ornaments, and emblems...

(Bourdieu, 1977, p165)

More recently, Gardner, in her studies of Bangladeshi migrants in London, has pointed to culturally distinctive ways in which age and the stages of life are identified (Gardner, 2002). In traditional agricultural societies the cycle of the seasons is internalised and incorporated into the everyday imperatives constituting duties and responsibilities. Representatives of institutions in the industrialised world frequently view migrants and refugees who are vague about matters concerning date of birth and age with routine suspicion on the assumption that these are basic components of personal identity that everyone should know. Apparent confusion about one's age is often seen as evidence of evasiveness and deception and may undermine claims for asylum. Thus, while the importance given to the measurement of age by calendar years is influenced by culture, for refugee children it represents a critical interface in which cultural norms may be substantively challenged.

Normatively oriented research focusing on life stages may also be seriously limiting in paying scant regard to the way in which subjects make sense of their lives. The sociologist Ken Plummer, for example, contrasts what he terms, '"objective" or scientific accounts of life stages which track early childhood through phases of Oedipal traumas, mirror stages, attachment etc., and on to the adult stages – of loss, despair, trust, hope, wisdom etc.', with what he views as a potentially more fruitful approach focused on 'tapping into some broad metaphorical images through which people come to develop their own sense of how their lives develop – the narratives of life patterns' (Plummer, 2001, p192). He suggests a range of narratives with contemporary currency in the West as having progressive global influence. One common form is what he terms the 'childhood fix narrative', which places a great deal of emphasis on the influence of experiences in early childhood. The narrative is 'told in a linear, sequential fashion which implies that life is a cumulative sequence of causes' (ibid., p193). Childhood experiences are treated as determining factors that shape the adult world. This type of narrative can be seen as underpinning a significant body of literature on refugee children which focuses on what Eastmond has described as the 'refugee curve' whereby the condition of refugees is described in terms of cumulative traumatic experiences originating in countries of origin and compounded through the experiences of flight and reception, and possibly subsequent deportation (Eastmond, 1998).

Authors such as Lillian Rubin highlighted problems with this approach:

The idea that what happens to a child in those early years in the family determines the future is much too simple. It assumes, first, that the child is a passive receptacle; second that the experiences of early childhood inevitably dwarf everything that happens afterwards. In reality, however, how the child handles those early experiences makes a difference in the outcome, as does what happens in the years ahead...too much intervenes between infancy and adulthood for the experience in the family alone to govern how a life will be lived.

(Rubin cited in Plummer, 2001, p193)

One particular approach identified in the research literature that relates this 'sense making' as having a positive impact on mental health and well-being involves engagement and political participation. Lynne Jones, a child psychiatrist who undertook extensive research on the experiences of children in the Bosnian war, points to credible evidence linking political participation to improved mental health outcomes in prolonged and 'low intensity' conflicts in Palestine and South Africa. However, the complexity of the field is illustrated by the fact that this did not accord with Jones' experiences of children in Bosnia where a quest for meaning, for making sense of the conflict, was accompanied with poorer mental health outcomes. She draws on evidence suggesting that children who do not seek explanations of catastrophic events and are prepared simply to take a position that they 'don't know' may be more mentally healthy (Jones, 2004, p230).

The fundamental idea expressed here that people could transcend extremely challenging early experiences and lead fulfilling and happy later lives presents a significant challenge to established norms embedded in a range of therapeutic approaches. In the present context, it draws attention from a conception of refugees as victims reeling from the impact of successive traumatic experiences, towards a nuanced and more complex picture which, while not underplaying the impact of traumatic events, considers refugee children as having the potential to mitigate the impact of events through personal and collective strategies. The emphasis, in short, is shifted from a paradigm of vulnerability to one of resilience. This raises questions not simply of the additive effects of traumatic events on refugees, but of the strategies that may be used by refugees to cope with adversity. More broadly, it suggests a preoccupation not only with the impact of political, economic and social factors, but also with the role of human agency. Of overriding concern here is the importance of a shift from a view of refugee children as largely passive victims of external events, to one that examines the linkages between externalities and individual and collective responses. Following Plummer, it implies an orientation towards understanding the ways in which people make sense of their lives, including the ways in which they may incorporate and transform individual and collective representations of themselves and their predicaments.

Conclusion

A range of theoretical approaches has been identified that are pertinent to an understanding of the position of refugee children. I argue that it is appropriate to view alternative approaches not as essentially better or worse than each other but as crucially related to the central research questions that may be posed. For example, the theoretical orientations identified by Castles and Miller have particular relevance to determinants and motivations for migration and its demographic characteristics. Within these capacious theoretical frameworks (push/pull, historical-structural, migration system, transnational) there is scope for the engagement of a range of disciplinary perspectives. For example, migration systems theories could be informed by macro-level studies of political economy augmented perhaps by ethnographic work examining the social and cultural linkages between migrants. It is possible to see the benefits of multi-level approaches within other contexts such as push-pull and transnational theories. For example, as push/pull theories are linked to the exercise of rational choice, it is highly relevant to examine them through research on processes of decision making, perhaps through small scale in-depth analysis of the decision to migrate among migrant communities or through larger scale quantitative and questionnaire-based studies.

The Foucauldian studies referred to here address somewhat different, episte-mologically oriented questions. They point towards examination of the social, political and historical contexts in which categories, such as 'refugee', 'asylum seeker' and 'illegal immigrant' emerge, are sustained and transformed. The con-cern is with examination of how objects of knowledge are generated and the human sciences that inform and sustain technologies of government. It is also, as we have noted, with the way in which people are the subjects of these technolo-gies and the impact this has on their sense of self and the way in which they conduct themselves. This is not, as we have noted, simply a matter of passive acceptance, but also of interpretation and reinterpretation, strategic responses and, in some contexts, resistance. All of these practices come within the sphere of governmentality as elaborated by a range of Foucauldian scholars, including spe-cialists on refugees and migration referred to above. A further contribution these studies make is to fix their gaze firmly on, and offer a theoretical and method-ological framework for, examining the interaction between migrants and national and international agencies. Their sphere of inquiry is thus not fundamentally dichotomised between government policy and procedures and the forms of knowledge that support them on the one hand, and migrant and refugee groups on the other. Malkki and Ong's work is particularly notable for the attention paid to the subjects of governmentality and epistemological processes of subject making.

As suggested, a related theoretical strand highly relevant to the present study is the emphasis on children's agency. As James and James have argued, within the social space of childhood, children are

> not just social actors playing a multitude of roles in relation to the increas-ing range of adults with whom their lives mesh as they move through their own childhoods towards adulthood. They are also social agents in that they shape those roles, both as individuals and as a collectivity, and they can create new ones that alter the social space of childhood to be inherited by the next generation.
>
> (James and James, 2004, p213)

As we have noted, this emphasis is not confined to studies focusing on children in the industrialised world, but also pervades research on children in the developing world and refugee children. Even in circumstances of extreme adversity, the latter are shown to frequently exercise agency in interpreting their circumstances and in responding strategically to them. The emphasis on agency is not to deny the impact of the adverse social circumstances in which children exist, but to encourage attention to be directed at the ways in which these circumstances are interpreted and navigated.

In the light of the above, an outline of an approach towards the study of refugee children may be tentatively drawn for an integrated approach that ideally recognises the following components:

1 Reflect the interrelationship between macro, meso, and micro levels and draw on a range of methodological tools and disciplines to illuminate this interrelationship.
2 Identify the structural constraints facing children, and specifically the role of social, economic and political factors.
3 Include analysis of the ways in which children respond to these external constraints, the ways in which they make meaning of their lives and develop strategies to cope with their circumstances.
4 Critically examine the social, political and historical contexts in which salient categories; childhood, refugees, asylum seekers, undocumented migrants etc. emerge, their practical impact and their impact on refugee children's subjectivities.

The following chapters attempt to reflect this integrated approach within the context of domains such as borders and the reception of refugee children, mental health, education and special programmes. This will indicate key challenges for academic researchers, policy makers and practitioners, and point to strategies for the development of social care services in the area.

3   Children at borders

This chapter focuses on the position of children seeking to enter industrialised countries as asylum seekers or undocumented migrants. The focus of the chapter is on borders in Southern Europe where thousands regularly attempt to cross from Africa or from the Middle East and South East Asia and the subsequent passage of refugees through parts of Northern Europe. For many, Southern Europe is but a further stepping stone in a journey to Northern Europe and, possibly, North America. Here we examine the struggles many would-be refugees endure to seek to enter Europe and the practices of deterrence that aim to exclude them. Within this broad context, the particular practices directed towards children at borders are examined.

One small step...

Within an international context, borders are, put most simply, places where people pass from one country to another. They are geographically situated places that demarcate the end of one state's territory and another's beginning. Ullrich Kockel has highlighted the material nature of borders in providing a conceptual distinction between borders, frontiers and boundaries, '*Frontier* refers to an interface area between different cultural systems; *boundary* means any cultural, political or administrative delimitation; *border*...denotes the more or less material expressions of boundaries between nation states' (Kockel, 1999, p7). Borders are often physically unremarkable, at first glance consisting of a few checkpoints and administrative buildings articulating only a circumscribed functionality. However, this façade is misleading as borders represent the convergence of a range of mechanisms of government, and apparently routine procedures of checking passports and goods disguise an intricate range of regulations and procedures that reflect fundamental and pervasive concerns regarding national sovereignty and security. Underpinning the visible practices at borders are a range of technologies of government, from precise criteria and procedures for entry, to elaborate systems of surveillance and a network of staff, from police and immigration officers to customs and welfare officers.

The positioning of borders and the technologies of government contained within them are reflective of the relationship between the states whose territories converge on the border and their positioning within multi-national alliances. For example, at the time of writing, many national borders *within* the European Union, and particularly those between countries that are part of the Schengen Agreement, are extremely porous, with little or no checks. By contrast, the external borders of the EU are heavily policed and would-be migrants, without access to the necessary papers, often feel driven to take life-threatening measures to enter the EU. Once within Schengen countries, movement from one country to another is relatively easy, provided the migrant has the financial means to undertake the journey.

There are parallels here with the border between Mexico and the United States, through which considerable numbers of would-be migrants from Latin America attempt to pass on a daily basis. It is intensively policed, with an extensive network of surveillance. However, despite these restrictions, the number of people entering the US and Europe continues to grow. In the US, the INS estimated that 7 million unauthorised immigrants 'were living in the United States in January 2000 and that on average this populace grew by about 350,000 per year from 1990 to 1999' (Inda, 2006, p163). The economic challenges facing irregular migrants is often considerable, however, and the movement from one place to another can often only be achieved through periods of working illegally and attempting to save sufficient money to continue the journey (Yaghmaian, 2005).

For refugees, borders evoke widely different responses depending on the context in which they arrive. For those who have entered legally as part of a quota of refugees already accepted by a host country, the border may evoke an emotional response reflective of a passage from one phase of life to another, blending nostalgia with apprehension and excitement. For those in the process of fleeing persecution, the border may be approached as a site of potential sanctuary where the persecutory forces are unable to enter. However, within this context it also may evoke feelings of acute anxiety owing to uncertainty as to whether the refugee will be allowed to cross and the potential harassment he or she may face. As Homi Bhabha has observed, 'The globe shrinks for those who own it, but for the displaced or dispossessed, the migrant or refugee, no distance is more awesome than the few feet across borders and frontiers' (cited in Gregory, 2004, p257). The border, which may have been a sole symbol of hope sustaining dangerous and arduous journeys, may itself turn out to be a dangerous place and the point at which all hope vanishes. The potential for this complete loss of hope is acutely evoked by the death of Walter Benjamin in 1940, while attempting to flee from the Nazis.

> In September, in the company of a small group, he reached the Spanish border with what he assumed to be the proper papers, but they were told at the last moment that they couldn't proceed. That night...Benjamin took a lethal dose of morphine. The next day, the border guard, not unmoved by the suicide, allowed the rest of the group to proceed.
>
> (Buck-Morss, 1977, p162)

For those who enter clandestinely, of course, the border presents itself as a significant barrier to meeting one's goal and one that may call on all one's physical energy and intelligence to circumvent. Those seeking a passage across the Mediterranean from North Africa to Europe often seek the support of smugglers to provide small crafts that can navigate across the waters undetected by border patrols. These journeys are notoriously precarious with many of the crafts barely seaworthy and often seriously overcrowded. Many of the people who attempt these journeys perish en route or suffer serious injury and mental and physical exhaustion.

It is, given its clandestine nature, difficult to estimate the number of undocumented migrants who attempt to cross the Mediterranean Sea. In 2002, Greek, Italian and Spanish authorities along the countries southern borders intercepted a total of some 35,000 migrants. On the basis of these border apprehensions, the International Centre for Migration Policy Development estimates that some 100,000 to 120,000 irregular migrants cross the Mediterranean each year, with about 35,000 coming from sub-Saharan Africa; 55,000 from the south and east Mediterranean and 30,000 from other (mainly Asian and Middle Eastern) countries (Lutterbeck, 2006, p61). Available evidence suggests that these people are not so much 'duped' by unscrupulous traffickers in terms of the dangers they face, but have made a rational decision to make the crossing despite the considerable risks, as they see the chance of getting to Europe as preferable to a life of persistent danger and desperate poverty in their own countries.

From North Africa

In considering the perils faced in attempting to cross into Europe by sea, it is important not to underestimate the hardships would-be migrants have endured in travelling from countries in sub-Saharan Africa to North Africa. Commenting on the situation of refugees in Cairo, Caroline Moorehead describes graphically and poignantly a catalogue of bureaucratic insensitivity and incompetence, detentions and brutality. To take one of several examples, she describes the situation of 'Mustafa' a boy from Liberia who had seen his first killing at the age of 11 'a cousin beaten to death in front of him when he failed to answer questions from rebel soldiers'. As he had the same surname as a rebel leader fighting government forces, he was regarded with suspicion and members of his family were gradually captured and killed. He himself was picked up, beaten and questioned and, fearing for his safety, he was picked up by a family friend and smuggled from Monrovia to Cairo at the age of 17. Moorehead describes his initial experiences in Cairo as follows;

> Mustafa spent three weeks in an Egyptian cell behind a police station in the spring of 2002. He was given only water for the first five days and kept permanently blindfolded. He was not allowed to use the lavatory. He was also slapped and kicked, something he made little of, being accustomed to physical brutality. In Cairo, prisoners call the room set aside in prisons and police stations for questioning and physical brutality 'the freezer'. Mustafa was not subjected to the electric shocks given to many taken into detention, but when they took off his blindfold after five days they put him into a small cell and left him there. It was not empty; on the contrary, it held about fifty people. There was no room for the prisoners to do anything but stand. They took it in turns to sit down.
>
> (Moorehead, 2005, p13)

Mustafa was eventually released and the reasons for his arrest and imprisonment were never explained, save for a rumour going round the Liberian community that Liberians were suspected to be Israeli spies owing to the rebel leader Charles Taylor's statement of support for the then Israeli leader Ariel Sharon.

As demonstrated in this example the precariousness of the situation may be exacerbated by local interpretations of international events, on the basis of which specific groups of refugees are targeted. The picture presented here of refugees living a liminal existence, seeking to survive on a day-to-day basis, watching and waiting for opportunities to secure their passage to Europe, while subject to the vagaries of randomised police action, is a common scenario, not only among refugees in North Africa but elsewhere on the globe. This modus operandi has some parallels with what Pedrazzini and Sanchez, on the basis of their fieldwork on the streets of Caracas have referred to as the 'culture of urgency' which Castells has described as 'the idea that there is no future, and no roots, only the present. And the present is made up of instants, of each instant. So life is lived as though each instant were the last one...' (Castells, 2000, p164). However, for these young migrants there is a transcendent goal that sustains them to go through the harsh immediacy of their everyday existences, the vision and goal of a life worth living in another place.

A passage to Italy

Italy's extensive coastline of over 7,000 kilometres has made it a particular target for migrants and refugees from Africa, Central and Eastern Europe and the Middle East. In the mid-2000s, 'it is the first country of arrival for more asylum seekers than any other of its European Union partners' (Moorehead, 2005, p55). According to official data, about 80,000 migrants and asylum seekers reached Italy by sea between the beginning of 2001 and June 2005. Moorehead records that up until the 1990s, influxes of migrants were generally responded to on a case-by-case basis, generally with leniency. However, following a series of landings through the 1990s of Albanians, Yugoslavs and Kurds, official attitudes hardened.

In a 2006 report, Amnesty International identified the following as risks of human rights violations affecting this group:

- refoulement to countries of origin or transit countries where individuals could face persecution and other serious human rights violations
- collective expulsions
- discriminatory access to asylum procedures
- unfair and inadequate identification procedures including age assessments
- procedures of adoption of expulsion orders and modalities of forcible return not in line with international human rights standards
- detention practices that fall short of international standards
- disregard of the obligations, prohibitions and standards concerning vulnerable groups.

(Amnesty International, 2006)

The 1998 Consolidated Law was the first comprehensive law in the field of immigration and has been the subject of increasingly restrictive application, being modified in 2002 by Law 189/02, commonly referred to as the Bossi-Fini Law. The law provided for the establishment of 'holding' centres, called centres of temporary stay and assistance – Centro di Permanenza Temporanea e Assistenza (CPTAs). In the introduction to a substantial report into their role and functioning, Amnesty International describe them as follows:

> Each year thousands of foreign nationals in Italy, some of them asylum seekers, are subject to expulsion or refusal-of-entry orders. These orders are issued on grounds of illegal, or attempted illegal entry to, or illegal residence in Italy, and the majority currently require that the people concerned be escorted to the border by law enforcement officers and expelled from the territory. While awaiting their removal from Italy these individuals are deprived of their liberty and detained in 'temporary stay and assistance centres', where they may be held for up to a maximum of 60 days, until the orders can be carried out, or the maximum detention limit is reached.
>
> (Amnesty International, 2005b, p1)

The conditions within these centres have been the subject of considerable concern, not only expressed by Amnesty International but also by lawyers, doctors, local NGOs, pastoral workers, members of the Italian parliament and international bodies such as UNHCR and the Council for Europe. Amnesty records that in May 2005 representatives of four Italian police unions made public statements expressing concern about various aspects of the situation in the CPTAs (2005b, p3). Human Rights Watch refer to the experiences of one Italian journalist who gained access to the Lampedusa camp in Sicily:

> The most detailed description comes from the Italian journalist Fabrizio Gatti, who spent one week in the centre in September 2005 by posing as a Kurdish asylum seeker. In his article published in the Italian magazine *L'espresso* on October 7, 2005, he described highly unsanitary conditions, including blocked sinks and toilets. At one point, Italian officers forced him to sit in sewage and kept him for hours in the scorching sun. On another day, Gatti reported, policemen forced a group of detainees to strip naked and made them and other detainees run a gauntlet. Gatti said he saw Italian police strike some of the detainees, and subject others to lewd and abusive behaviour in front of children.
>
> (Human Rights Watch, 2006)

The 2002 law also had the effect of decentralising recognition of refugee status to border areas through the establishment of Identification Centres (Centri di Identificazione) which allows for the 'generalised detention during the entire asylum procedure of asylum seekers arriving irregularly' (Amnesty International, 2006). The legislation did not come into effect until April 2005 and at the time of writing is being gradually introduced. However, although law and policy specifies provision for distinctive types of centres, in practice there is a blurring between the specified functions. A number of the identification centres have been converted from what were previously open first reception centres (centri di prima accoglienza), or constructed adjacent to such centres or to CPTAs, suggesting the formation of multi-purpose facilities combining the tasks of assessment, detention and expulsion. Since 2002 several existing centres have been used as de facto detention centres holding families with children for unspecified periods of time. The process of decentralisation allows the provincial head of government to entrust the management of the centre, by contract, to local, public or private authorities operating in the field of assistance to asylum seekers or to migrants, or in the field of social work. The law directs that unaccompanied minors should not be detained in identification centres and that attention should be paid to the particular needs of children, the disabled, pregnant women and those who have been persecuted in their place of origin. These provisions are in line with the requirements of the European Commission directive on the minimum standards for the reception of asylum seekers (EC, 2003).

In principle, there is a clear distinction between identification centres and CPTAs. The former are for asylum seekers, either those who have presented in the approved way at the border and whose claims are being investigated, or for those who have entered, or attempted to enter, in an irregular way and have subsequently claimed asylum. By contrast, CPTAs are for those who are deemed to have no right to be in Italy and have been issued with expulsion or refusal of entry documents prior to them being forcibly escorted to the border by law enforcement officers. As such, they are de facto deportation centres where people are held while procedures are undertaken, for example, necessary travel documents are procured or where some emergency humanitarian assistance is sought prior to deportation.

The reception mechanism for asylum seekers in Italy has been the subject of sustained criticism both for bureaucratic inefficiency, with asylum seekers waiting between 12 and 24 months for a decision from the Central Commission, and on the grounds that, while waiting, they have little or no means of sustaining themselves and no access to health care. According to a 2005 report by the International Federation for Human Rights, the failings of reception procedures are made up for

> by a great many reception solutions of a charitable nature providing...stable lodgings (such as Caritas, the Jesuit Refugee Service, many local religious missions) or activist lodging ('self-managed' squats, 'social centres'), or lodging programmes directly managed or financially assisted by certain municipalities.
>
> (IFHR, 2005, p9)

Despite the efforts of charitable bodies, in practical terms it is extremely difficult for asylum seekers to pursue their claims.

The International Fact Finding Mission undertaken by the International Federation for Human Rights did note some potential for improvement through the establishment of Territorial Commissions in seven localities with the power to grant refugee status. These were established in proximity to the various identification centres referred to above. However, the decentralisation of the process was not without real or potential problems such as disparities in processes between different commissions, and the training and resources available to them. Furthermore, the decentralisation of decision making brought legal processes closer to the local authority and personnel who were involved in the process of detention, the latter being represented on the Commissions.

The granting of refugee status involved the local authority taking responsibility for reception and integration with attendant resource implications. The IFHR also expressed concern that, 'there can be no certainty that proximity to the place where, in fact, the people whose application is being examined are imprisoned and whose release is dependent on the decision, is conducive to the impartiality and independence necessary for hearing their application' (IFHR, 2005, p14). Furthermore, besides these localised disincentives, the chances of gaining refugee status were relatively slim. According to Moorehead, writing prior to the introduction of the Territorial Commissions,

> since this process can now take a year or more, many have left their designated addresses long before the summons, to disappear into Italy's vast black economy, or to drift northwards illegally into other European countries. Only 20 per cent of those who apply for asylum turn up in Rome for their interview.
>
> (Moorehead, 2005, p56)

As outlined in the 2006 Amnesty International report, while the legal position of asylum-seeking adults permits detention in some circumstances and limited access to benefits, asylum-seeking children have markedly greater protection. Detention of unaccompanied migrant and asylum-seeking minors is prohibited under immigration laws and minors cannot be expelled 'except for their right to follow their expelled parent or guardian' (Amnesty International, 2006). In short, this indicates that unaccompanied children will not be expelled but those who are in families may be. In terms of border situations, Italian legislation does not include specific measures to protect minors but all migrant minors, including asylum seekers and irregular minors, have in law the same rights to education and to medical care as Italian citizens. The rights and privileges of unaccompanied minors are complex, particularly with respect to the transition to adulthood at the age of 18. Those permitted to stay in Italy do so under a 'minor age' permit which they can convert into a permit for study or work only under certain conditions. They must prove that they have been in Italy for at least three years and been engaged in a project of social or civil integration for more than two years. Children who have not been granted refugee status who arrive in Italy after their fifteenth birthday, are not in foster care or lack certification of their 'integration process', lose their residence permit on the day of their eighteenth birthday and are liable for detention and deportation.

Amnesty International has raised a series of specific concerns with respect to migrant and asylum-seeking minors, many of these centring on the issue of detention. These include a lack of transparency with respect to the holding of minors in the different types of centres. Amnesty maintains that it has credible evidence concerning the detention of minors but is faced with official denials and the blocking of attempts to inspect the facilities. This included well-documented evidence that some 588 children arrived within family units from the Horn of Africa countries along with Kurds from Iraq and Turkey between January 2002 and August 2005. Amnesty believes that the numbers they have established are only a fraction of the numbers being held.

Concern has also been expressed that, contrary to national law and international standards, not only children within family units but unaccompanied minors are being held in detention. Amnesty reported credible evidence that 28 unaccompanied minors from sub-Saharan African countries had been detained between 2002 and 2005. It reported the following instance:

> Amnesty International has spoken to John who arrived in Italy as an unaccompanied minor, fleeing a life as a child soldier in his native country. After arriving on Lampedusa, he was taken to a detention centre and ordered to get undressed for a body check. He told them that he was only 16 years old, yet he was detained at the Lampedusa Centre for two days where he slept in a room with six adult men. He was later transferred to another centre in southern Italy where he had to share a room with 12 adults for a month. John eventually found accommodation in a reception centre for minors. However, five months after his arrival in Italy a guardian had still not been appointed to represent him.
>
> (Amnesty International, 2006, p5)

In addition to the above, Amnesty cites evidence relating to the detention of a further 275 unaccompanied young persons, many of whom they believe to be minors originating from North African and Middle Eastern countries. Further concerns related to the process of transfer, the living conditions within detention centres and the process of age assessment. Transfers, which in many cases lasted 12 hours or more, were undertaken with a lack of food and water and little or no information regarding the place of destination. Concerns about the conditions within the detention centres included specific issues relating to mobile houses which 'in summer are subject to intense heat and in winter to cold and wet', and which house many children under five years old (ibid.).

These examples are by no means unique to Italy. The detention of children is a feature of many asylum regimes within the industrialised world. It is notable particularly with respect to children who are routinely detained as part of a family group but has also been applied to groups of unaccompanied minors. Australia, for example, mandates detention for all non-citizens in the country without a valid visa. According to a recent study, 'this deprivation of liberty without any prior opportunity for legal advice affects all asylum seekers, including children' (Bhabha and Crock, 2007, p80). A major public enquiry into the detention of children in Australia resulted in changes introduced in June 2005 whereby children were to be no longer placed in immigration detention centres but released into 'community housing' arrangements.

Both the fact of detention and the conditions under which children are detained raise serious concerns with respect to a disregard for international human rights laws and standards. Perhaps most fundamentally the UN Convention on the Rights of the Child requires states to give primary consideration to the best interests of the child every time a decision concerning them, directly or indirectly, is taken. Article 22 states that children who are seeking refugee status, 'receive appropriate protection and humanitarian assistance in the enjoyment of applicable rights' and, further, Article 37 stipulates that 'Children shall not be subject to cruel, inhuman or degrading treatment'. Microanalysis of practices reveals the gap that often exists between laws, conventions and protocols and routine practice on the ground. The situation of refugee children often demonstrates a chasm between on the one hand the aspiration of society towards the positive treatment of children and the marginalisation and expulsion of those viewed as 'other'.

Spanish border zones

Spain's border areas are markedly contrasted and reflect some of the features of borders, boundaries and frontiers referred to above. To the north lies the border with France, which is porous and reflects the realities of the new Europe, offering freedom of movement and opportunity to its members. Besides sharing membership of the European Union, France and Spain are part of what has variously been described historically as 'Christian', 'Roman' or 'Latin' Europe (Kockel, 1999, p6). Travel between the two countries is now generally routine and easy.

The southern and eastern seaward borders of mainland Spain are markedly different both in terms of their contemporary symbolic significance and the nature and extent of the controls used to police them. It is probably not overstating the matter to suggest that this border zone combines symbolically all three aspects of the typology proposed by Ullrich Kockel. It is a border in that it is a material expression of a boundary between nation states, but it is also a boundary in marking a cultural and political delimitation, and a frontier in the sense proposed by Kockel, in that it marks an 'interface area between different cultural systems' (1999). Spain, like its partner EU countries across the Mediterranean, stands at a border of the European Union but also, at an international level, at the interface between the Christian and Islamic worlds.

The salience of this border area has been reinforced emphatically in the context of crude and pervasive characterisations of the international situation following 9/11. These often evoke Samuel P. Huntington's adopted and oft quoted phrase 'clash of civilisations' between the West and the Islamic world.[2] While ostensibly analysing the emerging relationships between Western and non-Western civilisations, most of Huntington's analysis is focused on the Islamic world as a notable 'Other' distinguished from 'the West'. Edward Said has identified the occurrence of 'undesirably vague and manipulable abstractions' such as the 'Islamic World' or 'The West' as emerging within specific historical contexts. According to him, 'They occur at times of deep insecurity, that is, when peoples seem particularly close to and thrust upon one another, as either the result of expansion, war, imperialism, and migration, or the effect of sudden, unprecedented change' (Said, 2001, p574).

The rhetoric and policy formulations directed towards the situation of irregular migrants at European border zones are replete with such dichotomising and essentialising language. Spanish border zones have become particularly acute physical manifestations of what, in another context, Stuart Hall has referred to as a dialectic of 'belongingness and otherness' (1992). The rhetoric of belongingness here is routinely evoked by the Spanish authorities in accentuating the position of Spain within the wider European community with which it shares common values and economic benefits. The evocation of a commonality of values implicitly underpins a stark economic argument that seeks to locate the 'problem' at a European level requiring European finance to address it.

Migrants trying to enter Spain are thus described as pulled by the attraction of a prosperous Europe and not specifically by the inducement of opportunities in Spain. The Spanish Prime Minister José Luis Zapatero spelt out this perspective in a statement coinciding with an informal meeting of EC heads of state at Hampton Court, England in 2005. In a companion article entitled 'Europe is the answer: only through closer co-operation can we secure the safety and prosperity of our citizens', the Spanish leader presented the problem as inextricably linked to the global economy and requiring an EU-wide response. He described the situation as follows:

> The tourists, workers, students and immigrants who arrive in Malaga, Barcelona, Bilbao or the Canary Islands are not arriving just in Spain. They are entering the largest area of freedom, democracy and social progress that exists anywhere in the world today: the European Union. This area, with a population of 453 million and 30% of the world's GDP, has some of the most powerful economies in the world and the greatest representation of western culture, tradition and history.
>
> (Zapatero, 2005)

The power and prestige of Europe is placed here in stark contrast to the positions of Morocco and the countries of sub-Saharan Africa. This is why, the Spanish premier continues,

> tens of thousands of people from across the world, seeking to leave behind abject poverty, war or repression, are knocking at the gates of the EU. Regulating the conditions of entry cannot be the exclusive responsibility of those who are near the gate. The border between Spain and Morocco is the scene of the greatest difference in per capita income between neighbouring

countries in the world, a proportion of 15 to 1. Morocco has calculated that its territory hosts about 40,000 people from sub-Saharan Africa who are trying to enter the EU. We are not facing a merely Spanish problem but a global one.

In May 2006, the Spanish Deputy Prime Minister echoed similar views in response to an increasing influx of migrants in the Canary Islands. Besides emphasising the matter to be of concern for the whole of Europe, she also outlined plans for the establishment of reception centres for migrants who were refused entrance:

> Spanish Deputy Prime Minister Maria Teresa Fernández de la Vega confirmed the EU would also help set up reception centres in Mauritania and Senegal for migrants who were refused entrance. She said the whole of Europe should take responsibility for the problem. 'It's clear that this is not just a problem which affects Spain, but one that concerns the whole of Europe. It's a difficult situation, which affects millions of people trying to leave their continent,' she said. 'We have to approach the migration problem from different angles: co-operation with the refugees' countries of origin, development aid and regulating the influx to Europe.'
>
> (Expatica EU News, May 2006, Brussels)

The above passages are notable for their political expediency, for the framing of the problem in European and global terms underpinning a request for the sharing of resources in response to a shared problem. Prime Minister Zapatero is arguably correct in his assertion that the immigrants in this context are, in general, drawn towards entering Europe rather than specifically targeting Spain. While, as a consequence of its growing economy, Spain offers the potential for casual employment, immigrants from Africa have few opportunities for sustained economic and social advancement. Many undertake short-term agricultural work, or attempt furtively to sell trinkets on the streets of cities such as Madrid or Barcelona as a preliminary to moving on to other European countries. Given the aspirations of the African migrants identified here the 'problem' is indeed one that should concern the whole of Europe. Beyond its more immediate political function, the above statement is notable for a stark juxtaposition between Europe and Africa. In a dichotomising worthy of Huntington, while Europe evokes Enlightenment values of 'freedom, democracy and social progress', Africa is associated here with abject poverty, war and repression. Africa as such is not only significantly weaker than Europe economically, but here is represented as its very antithesis in terms of social and political development.

Given this scenario, there is an implicit assumption that the numbers seeking to enter Europe are potentially limitless, calling for concerted action. It is notable that, while war and repression are identified as features of Africa, there is no further mention of the possibility that those seeking entry to Europe may be victims of persecution and in need of protection. Instead, the agenda for action defined here is focused on controlling immigration, countering illegality, fighting terrorism and promoting development aid to countries of origin. This perspective accords with the stark assertion made by Amnesty International that 'refugees are invisible in Spain'. It points out that asylum seekers and refugees are rarely referred to in statements made by ministers, the press or public bodies, with those attempting to enter Spain by its southern border being referred to as 'irregular migrants', 'without mentioning the possibility that some of them may, in fact, be fleeing persecution and grave violations of human rights' (Amnesty International, 2005a, p2).

Within this broader scenario, Morocco is viewed as a potential threat to Europe both because of the relative weakness of its economy and as a transit country for would-be migrants from sub-Saharan Africa. The country has long-standing relationships with a number of European countries with respect to labour migration and agreements were signed through the 1960s with Germany, France, Belgium and the Netherlands (Collyer, 2004). The country benefited significantly from remittances sent by emigrants. According to Collyer, Moroccans sent back huge proportions of their income; 'in the late sixties it was estimated that single Moroccans sent back between 80 and 90 percent of their salaries and a survey in France in 1972 found that 89 percent of Moroccans sent money back, the highest proportion of any migrant group surveyed' (ibid., p16). In 1985 it was estimated that total transfers resulting from North African emigration to Europe stood at US$4–5 billion (Castles and Miller, 2003, p127). A more recent study shows that, in 2000, an emigrant community of 1,669,738 Moroccans sent a total of the equivalent of $3,460,000 in remittances, with the vast majority of this money from emigrants in EU countries (ibid., p32).

Castles and Miller point to the interlinkages between, on the one hand the changing nature of the relationships between Morocco and Spain and the EU and, on the other, the development of irregular migration between the two countries. They point out that Moroccans and sub-Saharan Africans 'had long transited through Spain to points in Europe, mainly to France prior to 1973 and afterwards to Italy' (ibid.). However, Spain's adhesion to the Schengen Agreement in 2001 resulted in the imposition of visa requirements on Moroccan citizens, with concomitant pressures placed on Morocco to increase restrictions on the flow of migrants from the south. The freedom of movement within the 'new Europe' was thus inextricably linked to the imposition of external constraints. Drawing on the work of Belguendouz, Castles and Miller note that the imposition of visa requirements on Moroccan citizens coincided with the first pateras or little boats carrying migrants across the Mediterranean to Spain (ibid.). Cornelius similarly identifies the growth of pressure on Spain from its more northerly European neighbours and argues that it was only from the mid-1990s that the Spanish government initiated surveillance of 'hot-spots' for illegal immigration. He argues that the European Union 'have long regarded Spain as one of the weakest points in the EU's security perimeter' (Cornelius, 2004, p407). In the early 2000s efforts were made to control the flow of North African and sub-Saharan African migrants by developing partnership arrangements between the EU and a number of 'sending' countries. Algeria co-operated by increasing border enforcement along its long and porous borders with Libya and Niger, a major route through which migrants from sub-Saharan Africa sought to access Europe via Algeria and Morocco (Castles and Miller, 2003, p125).

The significance of the Spanish border zone doesn't end with the seaward proximity to Africa in the south. There are the Spanish-controlled territories of Ceuta and Melilla situated on the African mainland on the northern Moroccan coast. Furthermore, there are the Canary Islands, a group of seven islands off the north coast of West Africa, about 1,050 kilometres from the Spanish mainland. Ceuta and Melilla have been under Spanish control since the sixteenth century, a matter that is the subject of ongoing dispute with Morocco, which regards them as occupied territories. These cites have been described as 'duty free ports with significant military presences and economies largely dependent on fishing, tourism, trade with Morocco, illicit drug trafficking, and profits gleaned from the smuggling of undocumented migrants on to Spanish territory' (Gold, 2000).

While in recent history Ceuta and Melilla were primarily seen as profitable trading centres, recently Ceuta in particular has gained widespread notoriety as a point where desperate migrants attempt to cross into Europe. The town is located on the north coast of Morocco, 14 kilometres from the Spanish peninsula. It covers an area of 20 square kilometres and has a population of approximately 72,000 (Gold, 2000). Once in Ceuta or Melilla, those seeking asylum are legally on Spanish territory and, as such, should enter into the Spanish process for determining refugee status. In recent years very large numbers of people from sub-Saharan Africa have been identified attempting to cross to the Spanish enclaves. Moroccan immigration enforcement statistics, published for the first time from 1999, showed that in 1995, 444 sub-Saharan Africans were detained for attempting illegal migration. Five years later, in 2000, the figure had increased dramatically to 10,000 (Castles and Miller, 2003, p125). To counter the potential influx of migrants, Spanish authorities in 2005 sought to double the size of a three-metre high fence on its six-mile long frontier. The border zone was, in 2005, already 'equipped with sensor pads, movement detectors, spotlights, infrared cameras and patrolled by the Spanish civil guard' (Tremlett, 2005). The cost of these high-tech security measures was borne by the European Union (Cornelius, 2004, p407).

From the mid-2000s the Spanish border zones have been witness to a compelling and tragic human drama as African migrants resorted to increasingly desperate measures to enter the European Union, and the Spanish and Moroccan authorities introduced increasingly draconian measures to keep them out. The migrants try to cross en masse in groups of up to 200 in the hope that at least some will survive. One migrant said to the Spanish *El Periodico* newspaper, 'we go in a group and all jump at once. We know that some will get through, that others will be injured and others may die, but we have to get through, whatever the cost' (Tremlett, 2005).

Journalists have reported several thousand people living in woods around Ceuta and Melilla hoping for an opportunity to cross the border. While there, they lead the most basic of existences, with virtually no shelter and minimal amounts of food and water. Attempts by NGOs to help the migrants are reportedly hampered by the fact that they need government authorisation to work in Morocco and this is not forthcoming because the government does not acknowledge that there are migrants living in the woods (Moura, 2005).

For migrants, the consequences of apprehension by the Moroccan authorities could be severe. In October 2005, a reported 500 migrants who were trying to get into Ceuta and Melilla were rounded up and forced onto buses. They were driven 18 miles and abandoned in the Moroccan desert without food and water. According to *Guardian* journalist, Giles Tremlett, Moroccan authorities were eventually shamed into picking them up while 'more than 1000 handcuffed migrants were...being bussed south towards the border with Mauritania. Several hundred more were being taken north to Oujda, where they were being put on military flights to Mali and Senegal' (Tremlett, 2005). Amnesty International has reported a number of instances in which, following entry onto Spanish territory and the requesting of asylum, asylum seekers have been clandestinely expelled. According to a report from Médecins Sans Frontières:

> In November 2003, S.F., a man from Gambia, was detained by state agents who took him to the border fence with Morocco. Before expelling him on the other side, they tore up his documentation, including the appointment to formalise his asylum application. The next day, he was detained close to the fence by a Moroccan patrol and taken to Oujda, where he was abandoned in a desert area near the border with Algeria.
>
> (Amnesty International, 2005a, p18)

Amnesty cites further evidence of systematic clandestine expulsion in documenting the cases of seven asylum seekers who were expelled following a raid on their lodgings by the Spanish Civil Guard in December 2004 (ibid.). These expulsions contravene both international and domestic Spanish law, which require that no asylum seeker may be expelled until their application has been deemed inadmissible. The evidence deriving from detailed studies undertaken by a range of reputable NGOs presents a disturbing picture. It is notable in this respect that many of the nationalities identified by Amnesty International of those hiding in the woods around Ceuta accorded with countries associated with high levels of human rights violations and refugee numbers by UNHCR (UNHCR, 2006b). While it cannot be assumed that all of the migrants from these countries are entitled to protection under the provisions of international refugee law, it is certainly likely that a significant proportion of the asylum seekers would fulfil criteria for determining refugee status.

As increasingly severe restrictions on entry have been imposed on the Spanish enclaves in North Africa and on seaward crossings through the Straits of Gibraltar, more migrants have been attempting the hazardous seaward crossing to the Canary Islands. According to a 2005 report by Amnesty International, over the past four years over 30,000 migrants had arrived by small boat in the Canary Islands from North Africa, Morocco and Mauritania (Amnesty International, 2005a, p50). The 2005 Amnesty International report describes the process whereby migrants attempt the crossing from the shores of Morocco:

The small boats normally transport between 20 and 35 people on a journey that lasts on average 20 hours, during which they can hardly move for fear of these very unstable vessels capsizing. In addition, since the penalties for trafficking networks were increased in 2003, many of the small boats sail without their master and carry more passengers...the increased political and judicial pressure on owners has given rise to an increased risk of shipwreck.

(Amnesty International, 2005a, p52)

Since 2005 the position has, if anything, become more serious. Moroccan authorities have closed a route from the Western Sahara leading to migrants seeking to make a longer and more hazardous crossing from ports in Mauritania. Writing in March 2006, Giles Tremlett reported that: 'A Spanish hospital ship and patrol boats trawled international waters off Mauritania yesterday looking for would-be immigrants on a new and dangerous sea route from Africa to Europe that has already claimed more than 1000 lives' (Tremlett, 2006).

To attempt to stem the flow of people leaving from Mauritania, the Spanish authorities were attempting to set up a refugee camp at the Mauritanian port city of Nouadhibou. One of Tremlett's interviewees, a Nigerian priest who cared for migrants in the port, highlighted the symbiotic relationship between the closure of routes to gain access to Europe and the increasingly desperate measures to get in: 'If they close off Nouadhibou it'll be Senegal or Cape Verde islands they leave from next – even longer distances and even more who will die' (ibid.).

Children at the Spanish border

According to a recent report on the situation of refugees in Morocco, 'many asylum seekers, whose status is not yet legalised, are detained only until an adequate number of "illegal immigrants" have been collected (1–200), and they are then deported to the border with Algeria'. The author of the report goes on to assert that, 'some asylum seekers related that they had been subject to deportation more than twenty times: "Unless you can bribe your way out, they just leave you in the desert to die". These asylum seekers had all made their way back into Morocco' (Lindstrom, 2002, p23). The report also highlights a pervasive problem of racism, directed in particular against black refugees. According to Lindstrom this discrimination had particular effects on refugee children,

refugees asserted that their children have been subject to racism in Moroccan schools by both teachers and other students alike, because of the colour of their skin and the lack of fluency in French and Arabic. Some refugee children are significantly older than their classmates because of interruptions of (sic) their education, sometimes for several years, another source of significant discrimination.

Some refugees reported that they had not been outside of their house for three months because of fear of confrontation with the police and several reported that they had been beaten on the streets without provocation. According to one of the refugees, 'the Moroccans see no difference between a refugee and an illegal immigrant. All black Africans are perceived as taking their jobs, cars, women, what have you. They spit at you in the street, and they provoke you into a fight' (Lindstrom, 2002, p21).

While the above scenario relates to migrants and refugees in general including women, men and children, there are specific concerns relating to migrant and refugee children. A range of NGOs, including Amnesty International and Human Rights Watch, the latter having devoted a major report to the situation of migrant children on the Moroccan/Spanish border, has investigated these concerns. The Human Rights Watch report entitled *'Nowhere to Turn: State Abuses of Unaccompanied Migrant Children by Spain and Morocco'* is focused primarily on the situation of Moroccan children who cross the border with Spain on a regular basis. It documents the harsh, and sometimes brutal, treatment received by these children both directly from the authorities and from other children in contexts where they are offered little or no protection. The report describes how, every year, thousands of Moroccan children 'some as young as ten', enter Ceuta and Melilla driven by dreams of better lives in Europe. According to Clarissa Bencomo, researcher in the Children's Rights Division of Human Rights Watch, 'No one is caring for these children. Spanish officials violate these children's human rights in an effort to drive them back to Morocco, and Moroccan officials punish them for having left' (Human Rights Watch, 2002b).

According to a report from a regional conference on migration and unaccompanied minors held under the auspices of the Council of Europe in 2005, Moroccan children experience a number of 'push factors' leading them to attempt to migrate (M'Jid, 2005). The first of these is defined as the socio-economic context of the country in which 40 per cent of people live below or just above the poverty line. Figures from the Moroccan Bureau of Statistics indicate that the poverty rate rose 58 per cent between 1991 and 1998, from 13.1 per cent to 19 per cent, affecting 27.2 per cent of the rural population and 12 per cent of the urban population (cited in Human Rights Watch 2002a, p8). Official unemployment rates at the end of 2001 stood at 13 per cent, with significantly higher rates of 20 per cent unemployment recorded for youths aged 15 to 24. While the economic situation was particularly acute in rural areas it is hard to generalise, as there were high levels of poverty in towns. In the sphere of education there have been improvements in recent years, with relatively higher enrolment rates for both girls and boys in primary education. However, despite this, more than 48 per cent were reported to be illiterate in 2005 (M'Jid, 2005, p9). The most significant determinant of low school attendance is poverty with only 36.3 per cent of children from poor families going to school according to a 2001 World Bank Report (cited by Human Rights Watch, 2002a, p8).

According to Najat M'Jid, an expert on the clandestine migration of children, the socio-economic context prevents children from

> projecting themselves into a Moroccan future. The myth of the European El
> Dorado becomes their dream and migration to Europe their life plan, whatever

price they have to pay. These young people think they have nothing more to lose since in any case they have no life.

(2005, p10)

They are instead 'pushed towards other places by the economic and social impasse in which they find themselves' and 'their perception of the economic possibilities in host countries' (2005, p10). Human Rights Watch adds to this the influence of European television broadcasts and 'a regular influx of adult migrants returning on annual leave provide children with a window on the opportunities for a better life in Europe' (2002a, p9). The hopelessness of the children's situation and the tantalising proximity of a potentially better life elsewhere may thus be seen as the respective 'push' and 'pull' factors determining the children's actions.

As Human Rights Watch has documented on the basis of extensive investigations in 2001, for those children caught by the police, there was 'a consistent pattern of police abuse in both cities'. Unaccompanied children in Melilla 'were beaten, clubbed, and kicked during forced expulsions to Morocco, and then beaten, detained in unsafe conditions, and then released on to the streets by the Moroccan police who received them at the border' (Human Rights Watch, 2002a, p1). The treatment of the children by the authorities in the two countries stands in stark contrast to the undertakings made by both Spain and Morocco to comply with the Convention on the Rights of the Child. In the case of Spain, the Convention has been codified in legislation according to which unaccompanied foreign children should receive care and protection on the same basis as Spanish children, including 'the right to education, health care, temporary residency status, and protection from repatriation if repatriation puts the child or the child's family at risk' (ibid.). When unaccompanied migrant children are encountered by the authorities, the latter have the responsibility to place them under the care of the Department of Social Welfare (Consejeria de Bienestar Social), a branch of the autonomous provincial government. The department oversees the running of five residential centres in Melilla and one in Ceuta, the San Antonio Centre. The day-to-day operation of these centres is usually undertaken at 'arm's length' by NGOs.

In Ceuta itself, a new project providing medical and psychological assistance to around 150 unaccompanied and undocumented Moroccan children started in October 2002; it was closed in June 2003 because of lack of political will to work toward lasting solutions.

(Médecins Sans Frontières, 2003)

Besides reported abuses by authorities in both countries, the unaccompanied children were often placed at the mercy of older and stronger children within the residential centres. This is an account by Lutfi, aged 12, recorded by Human Rights Watch (HRW) researchers:

Sometimes the police catch me and send me to San Antonio but I escape. I never stay there long because the older kids hit you and steal your shoes...The officials at the centre don't do anything when they see the older kids hitting the small kids...If you have money the older kids take it from you and hit you at San Antonio.

(Human Rights Watch, 2002a, p13)

The HRW research describes the residential centres as being, far from places of safety and security, harsh and punitive environments. Instances are recorded of children being physically beaten by 'educators' who run the centres and the operation of a punishment cell for those who abscond. The catalogue of abuse documented by Human Rights Watch provokes a sense of outrage both at the specific instances of callous brutality and towards the broader institutional factors such as the absence of regulatory oversight of the authorities' practices.

As argued previously, host societies' responses to migrant and refugee children may be characterised as informed by two 'trajectories'; one that is concerned with the welfare of the child and is underpinned by a range of statutory instruments and codes of practice deriving from various national and international instruments, and a second that is concerned with the security of the territory. The latter is concerned with the control of populations and includes physical and legal barriers to entry, the avenues through which legitimate entry may be achieved and the processes whereby non-nationals are monitored when on the territory of another sovereign state. The welfare element is normally localised operationally and is the responsibility of local government frequently in co-operation with a range of NGOs or the so-called 'third sector'. Separation and, on occasion, conflict between these two trajectories is arguably a necessary aspect of maintaining refugee children's human rights. Where the welfare regime is as in this instance, in practice, merely an appendage to the state's security apparatus, national and international standards of care for refugee children appear likely to be eroded.

The situation of the Moroccan children crossing into the Spanish enclaves is generally different in character to that of accompanied and unaccompanied children who land in the Canary Islands and make their way from sub-Saharan Africa, and those generally placed in the category of 'refugee children'. Although they may be seeking escape from various forms of abuse at the hands of the authorities or of family or community members, they are not even cursorily considered as potential refugees. Thousands cross the border each year, only to be routinely incarcerated as a preliminary to being forcibly removed from the territory. Laws, codes of conduct and institutional procedures are regularly flouted giving the impression of a welfare regime that, in practice, denies its own responsibility for welfare and is entirely complicit with the security apparatus. Following interviews with Spanish officials at every level of government, HRW reported:

An utter lack of effective monitoring and enforcement mechanisms or procedures to ensure that unaccompanied migrant children received the care and protection to which they are entitled in domestic and international law. Time and again officials charged with monitoring, coordinating, and providing care told us that some other body was responsible for investigating and enforcing children's rights to protection, or that they relied on their subordinates to inform them of any problems or abuses involving unaccompanied children, although in almost all cases the subordinates were responsible for the abuses. Without doubt, decentralisation and lack of coordination among government agencies contribute to human rights violations against unaccompanied migrant children, but the core problem remains an unwillingness to acknowledge and enforce these children's rights.

(Human Rights Watch, 2002a, p37)

The above examples again point to the importance of a multi-level approach to the study of refugee children. Laws, codes of conduct, statutory instruments and local government policies and procedures were inventoried, constituting a useful checklist against which to measure practice, but practice can only be properly scrutinised through what, following Lipsky (1980), may be described as 'street level encounters' with refugee children and those who are responsible for their care and control. This suggests a complementary micro level of research that is concerned with the ways in which policies and procedures inform practice. The examples given here from Spain, Italy and Morocco demonstrate the serious gaps that exist between laws and policies and practice, while also pointing to the complex and problematic interrelationships between governmental agencies.

Refugee children at the French and Belgian coasts

For those who succeed in crossing the international border into the Schengen countries, they are likely to be met with suspicion and hostility, both by immigration authorities and by the general population. However, this was not always the case and the shifting of the public mood in Western countries has been identified as a phenomenon of very recent history. As the anthropologist Didier Fassin has remarked, the period after 1951 witnessed a growth in the legitimacy of political asylum: 'The "undesirables" became heroes for some, victims for many. They served as symbols of resistance to the oppression, as in Chile after the 1973 coup, or of the suffering of oppressed, as with the Vietnamese boat people 1978' (Fassin, 2005, p374).

Fassin goes on to assert that, 'in fact, until the early 1980s, refugees were the most legitimate figures within the implicit – and sometimes explicit – hierarchy of foreigners, and they thereby benefited from relatively privileged conditions' (ibid.). He identifies 1989 as a turning point in France owing to a dramatic increase in the number of asylum seekers and increasingly restrictive immigration laws under which asylum became one of the few legitimate 'avenues of access' for entering a country (Watters, 2001b). Asylum and economic migration became increasingly conflated in political discourse, leading to growing mistrust of asylum seekers and increasingly draconian measures. Fassin's chronology broadly holds good for the UK, where some popular tabloid newspapers stoked up public disquiet by persistently linking asylum seekers to opportunistic claims on the welfare system and threats to national security. 'Asylum seekers' became a term in everyday discussion inextricably linked to imagery of cunning and manipulative foreigners securing generous material rewards from a hopelessly gullible government. In response to this imagery, successive Conservative and Labour administrations in the UK sought to dispel the myth, not so much by offering countervailing facts about the benefits given to asylum seekers, but by showing that they were 'tough on asylum', and increasing restrictions both to entry and to welfare benefits.

Many of these clandestine entrants are children, particularly boys aged between 15 and 18. There is, of course, considerable debate as to the extent to which these children are suffering from persecution according to the terms of the 1951 UN Convention. What is routinely clear to those who have contact with these children and know something of their circumstances is that they are normally fleeing from dangerous and poverty-stricken countries where they feel they have little or no chance of living safe and fulfilling lives. Often the migrants see their choice in the starkest terms; either they escape to Europe and have some hope of a fulfilling life, or they will die in their own countries. It is for this reason that they are willing to risk their lives in crossing borders.

Fassin notes that, for a high proportion of refugees, their objective is not only to get into Europe but also specifically to reach the UK, a country with an 'almost mythical status' among refugees (Fassin, 2005). According to Derluyn and Broekaert, on the basis of research into migrants and refugees in Belgium, the UK is their 'promised land, as they perceive the UK to offer favourable employment opportunities, along with other attractions, such as better benefit payments, better access to health care, and better social conditions than other EU states' (Derluyn and Broekaert 2005, p34). The appeal of the UK lies in the broad perception that it is a place where a refugee can 'have a future' through receiving education and training and good opportunities for access to employment. Furthermore, refugees often also see the UK as more tolerant and just than other European countries and with better opportunities for those from diverse ethnic and racial backgrounds.

That would-be migrants view the UK in this positive light is not only borne out by the large numbers who daily risk their lives to get there, having already reached the relatively safe setting of the EU, but also in interviews conducted by researchers who have undertaken studies in the ports of Calais and Zeebrugge (Fassin, 2005; Derluyn and Broekaert, 2005). The conclusions of these researchers are supported by my own interviews with asylum seekers and refugees in the UK where I found perceptions of the UK as having more opportunities were widespread, along with a sense, often disturbed among those at a later stage of the asylum process, that there was more chance of asylum claims being dealt with sympathetically. However, it was notable that many of the asylum seekers I spoke to in London were very anxious about the prospects of being dispersed elsewhere, as they perceived the country beyond London as places where they would be 'more visible' and were more likely to encounter hostility (Watters, 2002a).

European ports offering the possibility of passage to the UK have, in the late nineteenth and early twentieth century witnessed the arrival of very significant numbers of people from across the globe. In response to the amassing of large numbers of refugees in the French port of Calais, the Red Cross opened a centre in nearby Sangatte in August 1999. Originally the centre hosted 200 people but the numbers had swelled to 1,500 at any one time by 2002 (Kremer, 2002). The French Red Cross described most of the people as having one clear objective – to reach the UK – on which they had pinned all of their hopes. The Red Cross estimated that, within two years of its opening, 5,000 people had passed through the centre, 80 per cent of whom were single young men (ibid., 2002). A high proportion of the young men were in their mid to late teens and would be subject to age assessment procedures when, and if, they reached the port of Dover, on the other shore. Behzad Yaghmaian, a US-based Iranian academic who followed the path of Muslim refugees for two years described the impact of the camp as follows:

> Sangatte was soon a legend. From Kandahar to Kirkuk, thousands of migrants took to the road with one goal: arriving at the camp and preparing for the next stage of their journey – moving to England through the Eurotunnel. During its short life, some sixty eight thousand migrants passed through the camp. Between August 1999 and December 2000, the Eurotunnel security intercepted around twenty-nine thousand people trying to leave for England at the Coquelles terminal. The migrants were handed over to the French police. Nearly three thousand were deported. The rest were set free.
>
> (Yaghmaian, 2005, p298)

Despite these significant figures, Yaghmaian appears to have underestimated the numbers passing through the camp from its opening in September 1999 to its closure in December 2002 with Courau, for example, placing the number at 76,000 (Courau, 2003). The closure of the camp followed intense pressure from the UK government, which saw it as being effectively a staging post to UK entry. In the run up to the camp's closure, enormous pressure was placed on the government by powerful sections of the UK media who argued that the Sangatte camp was symptomatic of a government that had lost control of Britain's borders. The conservative *Daily Mail*, for example, ran regular headlines such as 'Asylum: Yes, Britain is a Soft Touch!' in which the UK was viewed as being overrun by unscrupulous foreigners presenting themselves as asylum seekers as a route to exploit Britain's welfare system (Watters, 2001b).

The pressures to close Sangatte also increased within France. According to Fassin, momentum to close the camp followed the introduction of a right-wing government in May 2002 in the wake of a presidential campaign 'centred mainly on public security issues'. Fassin records that 'the first act of the French minister of the interior Nicolas Sarkozy, was to visit Sangatte and announce that he would close it by the end of the year'. The arguments centred on two aspects; firstly that the camp was a magnet for illegal immigration and, secondly, that 'it was shameful in a modern democracy to allow such an institution to persist' (Fassin, 2005). In formulating the argument in this way, the government sought skilfully to mobilise support from both those with an overriding concern with national security and those with predominant humanitarian concerns, the latter particularly 'speaking to left-wing critiques that reference the dark memory of German concentration camps' (ibid., p364).

The political machinations surrounding the camp have tended to obscure the fact that it was developed as a humanitarian response to a situation in which hundreds of people were sleeping rough without the most basic of requisites. The efforts of a non-governmental organisation were then presented as themselves a 'pull factor' for migrants and, further, the constitution of the camp was itself criticised on ostensibly humanitarian grounds. The story of Sangatte is thus illustrative of a 'double-bind' experienced by a range of welfare agencies working in the refugee field; the circumstances of migrants and refugees give rise to an imperative to act, but this action is itself presented as an exacerbation of a perceived problem giving rise to pressures to curtail it. An assumption associated with the granting of humanitarian assistance is that acts of kindness generate the risk of encouraging 'hordes' of refugees to descend on a country or locality. A further feature of governmental responses, illustrated by the example of Sangatte and by the earlier examples from Morocco, Spain and Italy, is the denying of possible refugee status. The contextualising of residents of Sangatte or those huddled in the woods around Ceuta under headings such as 'irregular migrants', 'undocumented immigrants' or 'clandestine migrants' is suggestive of illegality and a lack of entitlement. When one examines the countries from which these people are drawn, in the woods around Ceuta 36 per cent were from the Democratic Republic of Congo, 12 per cent from the Ivory Coast, 12 per cent Cameroon and 8 per cent Mali and Senegal respectively (Amnesty International, 2005a). According to UNHCR, a high proportion of the people staying at Sangatte in November 2002, possibly as many as 75 per cent were from either Iraq or Afghanistan. The Asylum Rights Campaign, a European Union working group has put the number of Iraqis and Afghans as high as 90 per cent of the Sangatte population in 2002 (ARC, 2002). Leaving aside detailed debate about the numbers, what is clear is that potentially large numbers of people in both contexts are from countries that are war torn or, at the very least, are the subjects of well-documented accounts of violent oppression. This suggests that there is a reasonable chance that a significant proportion have legitimate claims for asylum under the UN Convention and/or would have a case for protection under humanitarian criteria. Prior to the closure of Sangatte, this possibility was recognised and underpinned UNHCR's involvement in recording the status of residents. However, in large part, public debate ignores the possibility that those seeking entry to Europe may have legitimate claims and a culture of mistrust is pervasive. As Daniel and Knudsen have remarked, in the life of the refugee 'trust is overwhelmed by mistrust, besieged by suspicion, and relentlessly undermined by caprice' (Valentine Daniel and Knudsen, 1995, p1).

Developments since the closure of Sangatte reinforce the view that the camp was a symptom rather than a cause of the movement of refugees to Calais. At the time of writing, there are a number of accounts circulating of the build up of migrants at the port, sleeping rough in derelict areas and relying on charities and religious organisations for basic provisions of food and clothing. There were informal estimates of a 14 per cent rise in the numbers of refugees in Calais in 2006 with approximately 500 sleeping around the port at any one time, including approximately 40 women. As when Sangatte was opened, the bulk of the refugees were young men, many in their mid to late teens. Yaghmaian has graphically described their bare existence close to the gates to the port in which they seek to survive on a day-to-day basis, living hand to mouth and making furtive and desperate attempts to cross to England at nightfall.

An alternative route to the UK is through the port of Zeebrugge in Belgium, 10 kilometres west of the Dutch border. Visibly, it recalls the anthropologist Michael Taussig's observation that the old ports of wood and stone are no longer used or are demolished to be replaced with, 'concrete container terminals...in moon-scaped industrial sites' (Taussig, 2006, p98). Zeebrugge is a major European port particularly for the transportation of freight with nearly one million lorries passing through the port on an annual basis. The port is highly significant economically with approximately 34.5 million tons of cargo passing through in 2005 and no less than 10,000 ship moorings annually (port of Zeebrugge, 2006). It is a major route for imports and exports between mainland Europe and the UK with ongoing crossings to the east of England. The issue of migration through the port came to international attention in a dramatic way in 2000 when 58 Chinese migrants were discovered dead, having suffocated in the back of a Dutch-registered lorry intercepted in Dover. The lorry had passed through the port of Zeebrugge without detection. Less well known was the subsequent discovery in Wexford, Ireland of the bodies of eight migrants in a freight container. Again the lorry had passed through Zeebrugge and according to an investigation by the Irish police the migrants had arrived in Ireland 'by mistake' as they had intended going to the UK (Doherty, 2001). The horror of these incidents has had deep resonance on both sides of the channel and added impetus for port authorities to implement measures to detect what those working at port authorities euphemistically refer to as 'illegals'. Two researchers from Ghent University, Ilse Derluyn and Eric Broekaert, undertook an extensive study of the position of unaccompanied minors who were intercepted at the port between January 2000 and August 2004. The foregoing discussion draws on their findings published in 2005 and on interviews I undertook with members of the Shipping Police in 2006.

Derluyn and Broekaert's investigations included a study of 1,093 data files of unaccompanied minors intercepted in the port between January 2000 and August 2004 and participant observation between January and April 2004 of the processes of interception and reception. In scrutinising the data files, the researchers identified 899 unique persons who had been intercepted, of whom 113 had been intercepted several times. In broad terms, the researchers identified the following process:

- interception
- movement to a Local Police Unit
- identification process (evidence of human traffickers or smugglers)
- referral to the Belgian Aliens Office – decision on what type of document the migrant receives.
- For unaccompanied migrants, the following options were available:
  - leave immediately
  - leave within five days
  - not obliged to leave.

Belgium is a signatory to the International Declaration on Children's Rights under which the unaccompanied minors must be protected and cared for until they reach the age of 18. As a consequence, the police are required to contact a child protection officer and from 1st May 2004, the Guardianship Office which has a responsibility for ensuring that 'every foreign minor not accompanied by a parent or legal caregiver has to be a appointed a guardian, who has to take care of the minor in all aspects of life' (Derluyn and Broekaert, 2005, p51). There is a relatively clear division of responsibilities between the federal government and the Flemish communities in that the former were responsible for those who claimed refugee status while the latter were responsible for those who didn't apply, in this instance the vast majority of the children. The researchers record that, at the time of writing, the federal government had 499 places in reception centres for those applying for asylum, while the Flemish authorities had reception provision for 32 children who didn't apply. Put in other terms, there were more than 15 times the number of places for those who apply for asylum than for those who don't. This division was notable, not least for the fact that the vast majority of unaccompanied minors intercepted in Belgium did not claim asylum in Belgium. In the 899 cases investigated by Derluyn and Broekaert, only seven minors decided to apply for asylum in Belgium, a mere 0.6 per cent of the total intercepted.

This is an extremely low number and is not reflective of the broader picture of unaccompanied minors who become known to the Belgian authorities either through making a claim for asylum or being discovered by the authorities by passing through Belgian territory without appropriate documentation. According to UNHCR figures, 603 unaccompanied minors applied for asylum in Belgium in 2002 and 589 applied in 2003, representing 3.2 per cent and 3.5 per cent of total applications respectively (2004). This is still considerably lower than the total number of unaccompanied minors known to the authorities, 1,135 in 2002 and 955 in 2003, but represents a considerably higher proportion of the total. These figures do not, of course, account for the inevitable fact that there are likely to be considerably more unaccompanied minors than those who are known to the authorities, with many passing through Belgium undetected.

Other notable features of the group studied by Derluyn and Broekaert, were their age distribution, gender and countries of origin. Of the 899 files investigated, 837 were males and only 31 females. Over 90 per cent were between the ages of 15 and 18, 30 were between 9 and 13 years old and 44 were 14 years old.

The researchers recorded that the main countries of origin were former Yugoslavia (177), Afghanistan (167), Macedonia (106), Albania (96) and Moldavia (94). The other countries of origin in order of frequency were Iraq, China, India, Iran, Romania, Turkey, Sri Lanka, Algeria, Vietnam, Palestine, Nepal, Pakistan, Belarus, Sudan, Russia, Columbia and Jamaica. Although girls generally constitute a small proportion of the total number of unaccompanied minors, the proportion intercepted in Zeebrugge was notably small, comprising only 3.45 per cent of the total. By comparison, UNHCR estimated that, of the 9,130 unaccompanied and separated children seeking asylum in selected industrialised countries in 2003, 28 per cent were female (UNHCR, 2004, p6). The UNHCR figure is more generally representative of that for asylum seekers in Belgium as a whole, where 32 per cent were female in 2002 and 37 per cent female in 2003. The countries of origin also indicate a distinctive difference from the general position in the country where, in the years 2001–2003, the highest proportion of unaccompanied minors came from the Democratic Republic of Congo, followed by Rwanda, Albania and Angola. The high proportion of asylum seekers from DRC and Rwanda is reflective of Belgium's former colonial ties, a linkage that is observed internationally as a factor in explaining the flow of migrants and refugees to particular countries (Castles *et al.*, 2003).

The unaccompanied minors in Zeebrugge were distinctive in terms of the wide variety of countries from which they originated and in their clear unity of purpose; to get to the UK. The desire to get to the UK was not reducible to former colonial ties nor, it would appear, to the existence of strong established like-ethnic communities. The UK is not noted for having comparatively strong communities from the former Yugoslavia, Macedonia, Albania or Moldavia, for example. The argument that the unaccompanied minors were simply seeking to move to a place where the economic conditions were substantially better does not explain why they routinely risked their lives to get from one prosperous part of the European Union to another and time and again undertook perilous journeys over the channel. What was clear from the interviews undertaken by the researchers was that the young people had in the main a very clear aspiration – to get to the UK. As one minor commented in his interview with Derluyn: 'I would rather swim to England...I would rather be dead than to stay in this situation'.

They found that there was a general perception that they could get a job quite easily in the UK and that they could have a future there. More specifically, the unaccompanied minors saw themselves as going to England, and London in particular, and frequently asked researchers for more information as to what London was like and practical advice on how to ask for a job. Besides the idea that they would get a job, they had a sense of a more benevolent society in which they would build a future. As one unaccompanied minor remarked in an interview with Derluyn:

> What would you do if you were in our situation? If there is nothing in your country? Wouldn't you escape? And if you know that you can't stay forever in a certain country, like Belgium; that, if you are 18 years of age, you will be

sent back to your country. Wouldn't you then also want to go to England like we want to do?

(Derluyn and Broekaert, 2005, p51)

Beyond a vision of jobs and general benevolence, researchers have noted that unaccompanied minors and asylum seekers have usually little idea of possible difficulties they may face in the UK. As Derluyn has remarked,

> It was sometimes very astonishing how these minors lack essential information about legal procedures and provisions and the reception structure for unaccompanied minors, about their current and future possibilities, about possible dangers relating to their journey, about living circumstances in the UK, and so on.

(Ibid., p49)

In observing groups of recently arrived unaccompanied minors in Kent, London and Manchester, they exuded a sense that they had 'made it' and that the challenges ahead were relatively trivial. This gave rise to some frustration among the officials responsible for their welfare who found it very difficult to gain serious responses to the challenges ahead. In interviews, British social workers would point out to me the likelihood that the unaccompanied minors who had claimed asylum would be returned to their own countries when they reached 18, and their seeming oblivion to this prospect. Many of those in an early stage of arrival had a sense instead that this simply would not happen; that, despite day-to-day travails, an overarching benevolence would somehow see them through.

Interception and reception in Zeebrugge

As noted above, within Zeebrugge the port's Shipping Police unit is responsible for the interception of stowaways and initial reception procedures. In an interview with two senior officials from the Shipping Police in 2006, conducted by the author, they described their primary function with respect to undocumented migrants as one of ensuring their 'safety' and emphasised the importance of this function with reference to the tragic deaths of the 58 Chinese migrants in Dover. An enquiry in to the reason migrants risked their lives to get to the UK rather than stay in Belgium was met by the response 'Do you speak Dutch?', suggesting that the key 'pull' factor was the opportunity to learn and function in the English language. They later went on to elaborate that they wanted to get to England because of 'friends, language and jobs'. The senior officer said that they had intercepted 680 migrants in 2005 and they repeatedly expressed pride in the particular role of two police dogs in the process whose function was to sniff the containers to detect signs of human scent. The police emphasised how friendly and effective the dogs were and that they had received national recognition through being on television. The process of detection and reception was described in benevolent terms with explicit emphasis placed time and again on their function – to ensure safety. They made it clear that they did not want to keep the migrants in Belgium as they had no aspiration to stay there: 'They don't want to stay in Belgium. We do a procedure and they go on their way' (Watters, 2006).

During a fieldwork visit police showed me a demonstration of how the migrants were detected by the dogs by arranging for one of their colleagues to act as a stowaway in one of the containers in a vast container park. After a couple of unsuccessful attempts, the man was eventually detected. The door of the container was opened and the dog bounded up to the man who was hidden in the back. The police pointed out that the dog did not bite and was not 'threatening'. I asked how the migrants reacted when they were discovered in this way and was advised that they were not frightened, 'they are told to expect this' and even speculated that even those who were detected for the first time knew all about the dogs, and even jokingly added that they may have had advance photographs of the police and dogs who might intercept them. The accounts emphasised how routine and even ritualistic the processes of interception were in which all parties knew what to expect. It would not be too crude a characterisation to say that the police took the view that the migrants knew where they wanted to go, they did not want to stop them getting there, but wanted to minimise the potential for accidents to happen en route. Their overarching interest was in improving detection through the appropriation of devices such as CO_2 sticks and scanners and not in the retention of those they intercept on Belgian soil.

After they are discovered, the 'illegals' were taken to an annex of three rooms close to the police headquarters. The immediate impression was of the dilapidated furniture and lack of decoration. One room had two or three desks with ripped coverings and a few uncomfortable wooden chairs that looked as though they may have been discarded by a local primary school, while in another there were two bedsteads covered with thin and dirty-looking old mattresses and an old blanket. The walls were undecorated, grey and austere save for one which had a surprising and initially incongruous graffiti display that centred on the image of a frightened-looking young bald figure with bloodshot eyes. The police explained that they had involved the local primary school in this, as they 'wanted them to feel part of things'. The rooms carried an almost tangible atmosphere of fear and sadness and the image of the figure seemed strangely appropriate. A third room was used for filming, photographing and fingerprinting the 'illegals' and included some rudimentary equipment for these purposes. Thinking about the migrants' physical needs after a long and arduous journey I made an enquiry about washing facilities. The police advised that there used to be a shower but it wasn't practical to retain it. 'Who would wash the towels?' one policewoman remarked, drawing her hand over an imaginary pile of towels with a look of disgust. The minimal facilities did not include access to health care and the police experienced considerable difficulties in getting a doctor to attend to sick migrants. One migrant had recently arrived with an injured leg and the police recounted spending all day on the phone trying to get help without success. Within the resources available to them, the police did try to give intercepted migrants a cup of tea and a little food, supplied by the Red Cross, before they went on their way.

The administrative procedures undertaken in the room with the desks included the completion of forms aimed at identifying the background and circumstances of the migrant. They were asked, for example, for their identity papers and, if these were not forthcoming, where their identity papers were. A number of the questions focused on seeking to ascertain the exact route followed by the migrant and particularly how they may have been helped on their journey. One set of questions, for example, is aimed at identifying whether the migrant has had to pay someone for their passage, how much they had to pay, and whether they 'had to work for the services rendered'. The orientation is towards identifying the presence of people smugglers and tracing their activities. It is interesting that while the migrants were euphemistically referred to as illegals and were usually travelling without the required documentation, police work was focused strongly on cracking smuggling rings rather than taking further action against the migrants themselves. There was nothing in the forms that was oriented towards exploring humanitarian circumstances that may have led the migrants to leave their countries. Only one of 22 questions in the police schedule asked why the migrant left their native country, the bulk were oriented around establishing identity, the processes of travelling and the networks that may have been involved.

The police advised that if migrants asked for asylum they were told that they would have to go to Brussels to apply and they were given an address to go to. They said that they were concerned about the condition and well-being of some of the migrants and did advise them that this would be an appropriate course of action. There were some limited resources to give them assistance to undertake the 60-mile trip. Those seeking asylum were 'logged' but not 'put on record' on the grounds that, if the application were formally recorded, this would show that they had made a claim for asylum in Belgium and consequently they could be returned to Belgium under the terms of the Dublin Convention whereby asylum seekers can be returned to the country in which they made their first application for asylum. The police were exercising a 'light touch' towards would-be asylum seekers to minimise the chances of an asylum claim being formally made. Indeed the processes and physical environment appeared designed to convey the overall message to migrants and potential asylum seekers that there was nothing in Belgium for them and that they should get on their way to their anticipated destination.

As Derluyn and Broekaert record, at the end of the process, migrants were given documents either not requiring them to leave Belgium or requiring them to leave the territory in five days. The police advised that a normal practice was for migrants to leave the police station and go to one of several 'safe houses' dotted around the port. As a police video demonstrated, these were in fact derelict often rat-infested buildings with piles of rubbish and excrement. These acted as a base from which the migrants would routinely try time and time again to reach the UK. Of the unaccompanied minors studied by Derluyn and Broekaert, after the formal procedures had been undertaken, including the engagement of a child protection officer, the unaccompanied minors left the police stations with those they were intercepted with to plan another attempt to cross the border. As the police tersely summarised the situation, 'we do a procedure and they go on their way'.

Although for most unaccompanied minors the interception thus is not necessarily the conclusion of their attempts to reach the UK, it was, nevertheless, often a deeply upsetting experience. As Derluyn and Broekaert remark:

> Intercepted in the port of Zeebrugge, many migrants see their dreams (temporarily) shattered by the police, and most find it difficult to understand what is happening, why they are intercepted, how long it will take until they can leave the police station, and so on. Many are, therefore, also very suspicious: 'What does Belgium have to do with the fact that I want to go to England?', 'What does Belgium earn with this?'
>
> (2005, p42)

I was struck by the human despair that seemed to cling to the walls of the reception rooms. On scrutinising the walls more closely it was apparent that they were covered with scratched messages. A few of those I noted were, 'Fuck Belgium I want to go to England', 'I came here from Italy I want to go to England'. Some were poignantly resonant of despair, 'I have given up. I wanted to go to England but now I am going back to my country – Angola. It is too hard'. Besides messages in English, they were written in a variety of languages, notably Italian, and a range of languages from the Indian sub-continent. The police advised that Italy was a frequent stopping-off point on their journeys where they made some money to continue. It appeared, although impossible to say for sure, that some had spent months or even years in Italy to get sufficient funds to take the next step.

Derluyn also noted the ubiquitous messages on the walls, and recorded in her fieldnotes:

> I am sitting on the bed in the police station, together with an intercepted minor, looking at the countless names, dates, words and texts written on the walls of the room. Most are in languages I do not understand, but some are universal language: 'London', 'Fuck Belgium', 'England', Love: Life of pain – Oceans of tears Valley of death – End of Life'.
>
> (Cited in ibid., p44)

The writing on the walls expresses a need among the migrants to record their presence in their own way and to tell their story, however fragmentary, within a context that is, for them both confusing and disempowering. They arrive in the rooms often exhausted, hungry and in physical pain from their exertions. Contrary to the view that they have been well-briefed on each stage of the journey and the impact of interception, they are usually very confused and fearful. The writing on the walls represents an opportunity to literally make their mark on an environment that is both imposed and constraining and in which the only permitted forms of expression are through the police interviews and the bureaucratic forms. The environment, while not normally overtly hostile, does manifest a culture of mistrust frequently referred to in writings on refugees (Valentine Daniel and Knudsen, 1995). The interviews were oriented towards discerning inconsistencies and revealing the assumed criminal gangs that were facilitating the process.

I earlier posited an analytical distinction in the responses of countries and international bodies to refugee children as being discernable along two trajectories; what I have characterised as the welfare and the immigration control axes respectively. The examples at the Spanish and Italian borders suggested an overwhelming influence of the security/control axis, in that welfare provision appeared minimal and cursory and generally supported, rather than challenged, the rationalities of immigration control. Within border areas the lack of investment in facilities to ensure the humane reception of refugees often stood in stark contrast to the extensive investment in security measures, as graphically illustrated in the security complex surrounding Ceuta, but discernible in border areas around the globe, from the US/Mexico border, to Australia and the Israel/Palestine border. The ferocity of the border control generally reflects, but (particularly in the wake of 9/11 and the 'war on terror') is not simply reducible to, the extent of the income disparities between countries or economic blocks.

The analysis of the situation of unaccompanied minors in the port of Zeebrugge challenges a number of prevailing orthodoxies within migration theory and the sociology of welfare. The unaccompanied minors in Zeebrugge were from a wide diversity of countries, some associated with flows of refugees owing to war and persecution, for example Afghanistan and former Yugoslavia, and some not. Some of the children and young people spoke to researchers of persecution in their countries of origin; all of them emphasised the aspiration for a better life elsewhere. To categorise all of these children as economic migrants is to ignore the interrelationship between economic factors, war and human rights abuses. As Castles has argued, 'failed economies generally also mean weak states, predatory ruling cliques and human rights abuses' (Castles, 2003, p17). On the basis of the conclusion that asylum seeking and economically driven population movement was frequently inextricably linked, Castles and others have put forward the formulation of an 'asylum-migration nexus' to reflect this phenomenon. The migrants at Zeebrugge and those huddled in Calais and in the woods around the Spanish enclaves are representative of the complexity of this interrelationship. As argued above, given the range of countries of origin, the enormous risks undertaken in their flight from their homelands and the desperate conditions in which they live, it is reasonable to consider that a proportion may well have a legitimate case for humanitarian protection. However, this possibility is rarely entertained within a pervasive culture of mistrust that informs the processes these migrants are the subjects of.

As noted, a common characteristic of the migrants discussed here has been their strong desire to go to England. This very specific orientation challenges the view that they are simply drawn by the potential economic benefits of Europe. The range of the groups seeking to reach the UK suggests that the

presence of culturally and ethnically similar groups is not, for many, a determining factor. What does seem to drive the migrants towards the UK is the
prospect of not only getting some work but of building a life. A similar observation was made by the writer Caryl Phillips following a visit to the Sangatte
camp and its environs:

> whether economic or political migrants, these people's lives are broken and
> they are simply looking for a chance to begin anew. A chance to work, to
> contribute, to make something of themselves. To begin again at the bottom
> of the pile.

> (Phillips, 2001)

The examples cited here show practices in border areas as imbued with a culture
of mistrust, with operational procedures routinely predisposed towards a view of
the migrants as 'illegals' driven solely by the motivation of economic advancement. The examples also show a predisposition on the part of the authorities
towards a minimal, albeit sometimes severe, level of engagement with the
migrants. The fact that they are on their way elsewhere provides a useful pretext
for initiating only minimal low-cost procedures deemed as sufficient to meet the
most rudimentary requirements of national and international law. As Agamben
has argued, the migrants and refugees represent a form of 'bare life', at once
both threatening and repulsive to nation states (Agamben, 1998). While bureaucratic procedures aim to exclude, these operate in a context in which even the
most basic sanitary provision is eschewed. The migrant is viewed implicitly as
polluting to the body politic. In these instances there is no desire to incorporate
the migrants and exercise the intensive forms of social control and surveillance
recounted in a range of studies that have adopted a Foucauldian approach
(Fassin, 2001; Ong, 2003). Procedures are formulated and executed in such a
way as to minimise the potential for the state to have any long-term responsibility for the migrants, as in the case of logging, but not formally recording, their
desire to claim asylum, followed by the suggestion of a 60-mile journey if they
wish to pursue the matter further.

The maintenance of a bureaucratic 'light touch' is challenged in the case of
children where there are more robust national and international statutory requirements to provide protection and care. For example, Article 20 of the Convention
on the Rights of the Child, to which Belgium is a signatory, states:

1   A child temporarily or permanently deprived of his or her family environ-
    ment, or in whose own best interests cannot be allowed to remain in that
    environment, shall be entitled to special protection and assistance provided
    by the State.
2   States Parties shall in accordance with their national laws ensure alternative
    care for such a child.

3   Such care could include, inter alia, foster placement ... adoption or if necessary placement in suitable institutions for the care of children. When considering solutions, due regard shall be paid to the desirability of continuity in a child's upbringing and to the child's ethnic, religious, cultural and linguistic background.

(UN, 1989)

Within this context, Derluyn and Broekaert note, the police contacted a child protection officer. The officer made the vital decision as to whether the unaccompanied minor would be transferred to an institution or be allowed to leave the police station. It was notable that an officer was not contacted in no less than 121 cases and in 110 of these instances the minor left the police station without any measures being taken. As noted above, where the child protection officer was contacted, in 399 cases no child protection measure was taken and the minor was allowed to leave the police station. While the likelihood of measures being taken decreased the older the child was, nevertheless measures were not taken with approximately half of the children aged between 14 and 16 years. Derluyn and Broekaert record that, in instances where measures were taken, most (70%) were sent to a crisis reception centre while only 44 of the sample were placed in a specialised centre for unaccompanied minors. The small numbers going to specialist centres was, they argue, owing to the lack of places available in these centres. They suggest, furthermore, that the lack of care provided in crisis reception centres leads many to attempt to leave and to try again to reach the UK. A similar conclusion has been reached by the Belgian-based charity Child Focus that investigated the reception facilities provided to trafficked children. They drew a clear link between the quality and appropriateness of the care provided and the rate of absconding. According to the charity:

So it was that in 2001 some 255 files on missing unaccompanied minors that had been communicated to the Centre were analysed. The purpose of the study was to describe the phenomenon in general and the profile of the minors concerned in order to promote a more effective approach to the problem. The lack of appropriate reception structures for minors who are victims of trafficking in human beings was one of the crucial points brought to light by the study. In fact, by force of circumstances these young people are often taken into institutions for adults, which do not meet their needs...

(De Pauw, 2002)

The BBC amplified the charity's findings by reporting that a large number of children who had been placed in reception centres in Belgium were being targeted by 'vice gangs' and were being drawn into prostitution. They reported in 2002 that 'nearly 400' children had simply disappeared amidst increasing concern for their safety (Wheeler, 2002). This phenomenon has been noted elsewhere in Europe with the UN Office for the Coordination of Humanitarian Affairs, noting in 2001 that 87 unaccompanied minors had gone missing in Sweden. This report coincided with newspaper articles alleging that children from reception centres were being used as prostitutes. The UN Committee on the Rights of the Child expressed concern about children in Sweden, referring in a 2005 report on child trafficking to 'The high number of unaccompanied children having gone missing from the Swedish Migration Board's special units for children without custodians' (UN, 2005).

The 1995 report in Belgium of the Committee on the Rights of the Child expressed the following concern with respect to unaccompanied minors. The Committee was

> particularly concerned that unaccompanied minors who have had their asylum claim rejected, but who can remain in the country until they are 18 years old, may be deprived of an identity and denied the full enjoyment of their rights, including health care and education. Such a situation, in the view of the Committee, raises concern as to its compatibility with articles 2 and 3 of the Convention.
>
> (Concluding observations of the CRC 20th June 1995)

A notably more benign view of Belgium's performance was adopted in a later Committee report in 2002. However, the NGO Human Rights Without Frontiers commented that specific concerns remained about the treatment of unaccompanied minors:

> The group of unaccompanied minors stands out as one requesting special measures of protection. Despite the various activities, including a draft law on the establishment of special reception centres for unaccompanied minors and a draft law on the creation of a guardianship service, Belgium lacks specific regulations for unaccompanied minors, whether seeking asylum or not. The UN Committee on the Rights of the Child emphasised the need of establishing special reception centres for unaccompanied minors, of ensuring that the stay in those centres is for the shortest time possible, and of adopting the draft law on the creation of a guardianship system.
>
> (Human Rights Without Frontiers, 2003)

While highlighting specific areas for improvement, the Committee made no reference to issues of detention and deportation despite concerns expressed by Amnesty International and Human Rights Without Frontiers. The latter pointed out that, at the end of 2002, children under 12 were being held in closed centres while Amnesty International have highlighted specific instances of detention and attempted deportation, as in the following example:

> A teenager from Guinea-Bissau who arrived at Brussels airport in November 2003 and made an immediate but unsuccessful asylum application spent some eight months in detention centres for aliens. During this period he was subject to several deportation attempts. The courts twice ruled that he should be released, allowed to enter Belgian territory, and provided with a guardian and

appropriate care in an institution where he would be protected as a minor. The Aliens Office disputed that he was a minor, as he maintained, and eventually transferred him to the transit zone in the airport in July, where he spent several days without food and sleeping facilities. Following interventions and publicity by domestic non-governmental organizations and the media, the Interior Minister ordered the boy's transfer to an open centre for asylum-seekers.

(Amnesty International, 2005c)

These examples illustrate the complex interrelationship between a range of agencies involved in asylum processes. While these are drawn here from Belgium, they are illustrative of widespread tensions in the treatment of refugee children within numerous industrialised countries. As noted previously, a fundamental and pervasive tension exists between governments' humanitarian obligations under international and national laws and the political and practical processes involved in immigration control. In applying the complex aspects of law impinging on asylum seeking and refugee children, courts often find themselves challenging government policies and practices. An additional tension is implicit in the formulation in many states of two quite discrete areas of law,

> migration on the one hand and child welfare on the other...In general, migration law is adult-centred, and child welfare law privileges citizens, with the result that unaccompanied and separated children tend to fall through a series of significant cracks.
>
> (Bhabha and Crock, 2007, p61)

The examples cited in this chapter highlight the importance of going beyond a macro level in the analysis of practice with respect to refugee children. What I have referred to as macro-level analysis in this context includes the range of laws and policies that impinge on a given locality. However, an examination that stops at recounting the various statutory instruments and guidelines, can say little about what Lipsy referred to as 'street level bureaucracy' (1980). A micro level of analysis here points to the importance of directly investigating the actual living contexts in which rules and procedures are implemented, or ignored, and the impact they may have on those who are their subjects.

Moreover the cases outlined here demonstrate the role of civil society and, in particular, the range of national and international NGOs, in calling governments to account on the basis of salient laws and conventions. Their contributions to the field are wide ranging; from macro-level roles in the development of laws and policies, to intermediate investigation into the formulation of policies in relation to countries' adherence to legal undertakings. A critical aspect of this work is the access NGOs have 'on the ground' to the situations within which children are placed. This determination to examine circumstances at first hand underpins the wide-ranging criticisms of the treatment of children in the various contexts referred to above. Additionally, as the work of Derluyn and Broekaert has demonstrated, empirical investigation by academic researchers can document micro processes that reveal the application of policies and practices at 'street level'.

The representation of refugee and asylum-seeking children as situated in 'cracks' in the legal systems of receiving countries has a certain appropriateness in relation to situations in which asylum claims have been made. However, in many of the examples identified here there are processes of what may be described as *systematic non-incorporation*. The descriptions of processes within border areas of Italy, Spain and Belgium suggest that rather than being explicitly discouraged or denied the right to claim asylum, both children and adults are subjected to systems where the issue of asylum barely arises and, if it does, gives rise to almost insurmountable complexity. As such, these processes are suggestive of what Lukes in his influential typology has identified as a second 'dimension' in the exercise of power in which, rather than the site of overt struggle, power is exercised in a covert manner by taking some matters off the agenda (Lukes, 2005). This may be seen as exemplified by what immigration authorities characterised as their 'light touch' towards unaccompanied minors whom they believe to be passing through and destined elsewhere. Where potential asylum seekers were seeking entry to countries of Europe's southern borders, more heavy-handed mechanisms were often in place to prevent entry to the territory and, on occasions, to summarily expel those who did cross the border.

4 Unaccompanied minors

From ports of entry to a mixed economy of care

In this chapter the position of unaccompanied refugee children arriving in the UK is examined. The material presented here draws in particular on studies in the port of Dover within the local authority area of Kent County Council and in areas to which the children were dispersed. The focus here is on various mechanisms whereby children are categorised and placed in particular contexts of care specifically through processes of age determination and needs assessment. The regimes of care within which they are situated are examined in relation to their economic and legal determinants. These give rise to a mixed economy of care wherein service providers seek to meet often rapidly shifting legal requirements within contexts of severe constraints on resources.

A significant proportion of the refugee children who reach England pass through the port of Dover, a major port of entry to the UK. For many, as demonstrated in the previous chapter, this is the realisation of a dream that has sustained them on a harrowing journey that may have taken them half way round the world. As Dover is a sea port, adjacent to the European mainland, those who arrive are likely to have travelled for long distances by road, possibly stopping for long periods of time, perhaps months or even years, in intermediate countries where they have sought to generate sufficient resources to continue their journeys. The children who arrive are bedraggled, exhausted and, sometimes, quietly elated. The journeys have been undertaken at considerable cost physically, mentally, emotionally and financially and have been powerfully sustained by dreams and expectations of a better life elsewhere. From interviews with asylum seekers, these revolved around achieving a sense of safety and security in an environment that is not hostile and that supports their aspirations towards achieving an education and getting a job.

The port is located in the South East of England close to the coastline with France. Historically, it was a major point of entry and exit to and from England since the Middle Ages and a site of considerable strategic military importance. It was the port through which Richard the Lionheart departed on the Third Crusade in 1191 to quell the armies of Saladin and was a major site in the defence of Britain in the Second World War. In the past half century, the military significance of Dover has progressively given way to an image of the port associated with peaceful trade with mainland Europe and a burgeoning tourist industry. At the time of writing, Dover had annually some 15 million passengers passing through the port and 1.7 million lorries, making it the busiest sea port in the UK. It may be seen as a 'borderland' in the sense put forward by Clifford that it is distinct in presupposing a territory defined by a geo-political line: two sides arbitrarily separated and policed, but also joined by legal and illegal practices of crossing and communication' (Clifford, 1994). In the case of Dover, the line is far from arbitrary and consists of just less than 42 kilometres (26 miles) of seawater. For many asylum seekers, these 26 miles represent a final challenge to be overcome on their journey and may be the subject of repeated attempts, hidden in lorries crossing by ferry or through the nearby channel tunnels. As Derluyn and Broekaert noted, many of the children in Zeebrugge had been intercepted several times and will go on trying until they either reach their destination or give up through exhaustion or injury (Derluyn and Broekaert, 2005).

According to UNHCR figures, between 2001 and 2003, 204,870 asylum seekers arrived in the UK of which 12,400 were unaccompanied or separated children. In 2001 there were 3,470 applications from unaccompanied children, in 2002 6,200 and in 2003 2,800, representing 4.9, 7.4 and 5.7 per cent of the total number of applications received in each of the years (UNHCR, 2004). These figures draw on data supplied by national governments, but there is nevertheless an indication of the scrutiny that should be adopted towards these figures in that the UK Home Office figure for 2003 was 3,180 (Wade *et al.*, 2005, p5). The highest numbers of applications were then received from children from Iraq, Afghanistan, Serbia and Montenegro, and Somalia followed by China, Albania, Angola, Eritrea, Vietnam and Ethiopia respectively. Between industrialised countries, there is considerable variation in the proportions of the total number of asylum seekers who are unaccompanied minors. Between 2001 and 2003, the Netherlands for example recorded more than 40 per cent of the total number of asylum seekers from Angola, Guinea and China as being unaccompanied minors. No less than 66 per cent of Afghan asylum seekers in Hungary were unaccompanied minors as were 54 per cent of an albeit small number of Afghan asylum seekers in New Zealand. In the UK proportionately the highest numbers of unaccompanied minors seeking asylum between 2001 and 2003 came from Serbia and Montenegro (22 per cent), Vietnam (20 per cent), Albania (19 per cent), Eritrea (17 per cent) and Angola (14 per cent). In 2003 unaccompanied and separated children asylum claims constituted 5.7 per cent of claims in the UK, 3.5 per cent of claims in Belgium, 1.9 per cent of claims in Germany and 9.1 per cent of claims in the Netherlands (UNHCR, 2004).

It is difficult to assess the significance of these figures and, as noted in Chapter 1, numbers are influenced by factors such as the quality of the registration procedure and variations between countries in the age bands incorporated in the definition. Part of the explanation for differences may lie in variation in the routes taken by smugglers, in the varying channels of possibility or avenues of access that open and contract in relation to the opening and closing of borders and the enhancement of security apparatuses. Significant differences between neighbouring countries, for example, the Netherlands and Germany, may also be influenced by 'pull' factors such as greater possibility of a successful claim and a more benign asylum regime while claims are considered. These in turn are likely to change in response to pressures from national media and public opinion exerted on governments. The Netherlands, for example, from being considered relatively welcoming of asylum seekers is, at the time of writing, viewed as having one of Europe's tougher regimes. It is thus important that 'push' and 'pull' factors are considered alongside mechanisms of control that may be initiated by states in response to a perceived crisis in asylum seeking. As Walter Benjamin remarked when observing the emerging situation in Europe in the years leading to the Second World War, 'The tradition of the oppressed teaches us that the "state of emergency" in which we live is not the exception but the rule' (Benjamin, 1999, p248). In the contemporary industrialised world, the rapidly shifting and unsettled contours of law and policy relating to asylum seekers display a sense of perpetual crisis against which piecemeal and reactive policies are developed.

Within the UK there has been since the mid-1990s a plethora of new laws, policies and operational guidelines relating to asylum seekers, refugees and undocumented migrants. The sheer scale of the changes more than suggests a continuing uncertainty as to how to approach the broad issue of migration. Underpinning the raft of measures is a dichotomising of 'worthy' and 'unworthy', 'good' and 'bad' migrants. As in other industrialised countries, a central distinction is drawn between the 'genuine' refugee with whom the country is represented as having a long and creditable history of supporting, and those who are considered not genuine, and variously described, as already noted, as illegals, illegal immigrants, undocumented migrants, irregular migrants, bogus asylum seekers and, in Australia, 'queue jumpers'. A further tension derives from the fact that with declining birth rates in most industrialised countries, and increasing life expectancy, there is a perceived economic need, often in the face of general public hostility, to bolster those of working age to ensure that sufficient revenues are generated to support those entering retirement.

From the mid-1990s the British government introduced a wide range of measures aimed at deterring would-be asylum seekers. These included expansion of surveillance at borders to detect migrants by a range of mechanisms including dogs, heartbeat detector machines, carbon dioxide sticks and X-ray machines. According to a ministerial response on the 9th July 2002, an estimated 12 per cent of lorries at the port of Dover were subjected to one or more of these surveillance techniques (House of Commons, 2002). These measures were accompanied by an expansion of carrier liability regulations according to which companies who were shown to have transported illegal immigrants were subject to hefty per capita fines. According to a Parliamentary Home Affairs report published in 2001, in 1999 carriers were liable for fines on a total of 31,639 people including 13,660 who had travelled by air, 10,404 by sea and 7,875 by Eurostar trains that pass through the Channel Tunnel (HMSO, 2001b).

Further measures included the introduction of 'juxtaposed controls' referring to a process in which UK border controls were introduced on the territory of France and Belgium, and reciprocal measures introduced. Thus the decision as to whether to admit a person to the UK was effectively made in another country. If it was decided that the person should not be admitted then he or she was handed over to the French or Belgian authorities and vice versa, thus avoiding the country's own judicial processes. In welcoming these new measures, the Home Office Minister Beverley Hughes made the following remarks to the British Parliament in February 2004:

> With the measures we are announcing today, we are effectively moving our borders across the Channel – UK immigration officers will be able to stop would-be illegal immigrants even before they set off for the UK. We are making it more and more difficult for illegal immigrants to get into Britain...But we are not complacent. While there is no evidence of significant numbers of illegal entrants reaching Britain through other ports, we nevertheless are extending the use of high-tech scanning equipment along the north European coastline. We have to ensure we stay one step ahead of the criminal gangs who traffic people across Europe. And we are also continuing intelligence-led work to fight the people smugglers – with 27 organised immigration crime gangs disrupted and 24 facilitators convicted in the last eight months alone.
>
> (Home Office, 2004)

The tone and content of this statement is typical of government responses not only in the UK but across the industrialised world (see for example Inda, 2006 on the US). It combines an emphasis on the robustness of government interventions with an undifferentiated association of all those attempting to cross the border without the correct papers with illegality and criminality. The measures are described without reference to the possibility that some of the people who have sought to enter the country by unorthodox means may do so because they are escaping persecution. While government representatives routinely drew ethically resonant distinctions between worthy and unworthy migrants, at an operational level policies of deterrence routinely close the door on the possibility of any migrant entering a territory and making an asylum claim. The pride with which the Home Office minister refers to the measures taken to 'stop would-be illegal immigrants even before they set off for the UK', the so-called 'juxtaposed controls', represents an innovative approach and recalls a range of broader measures aimed towards the deterritorialisation of immigration control (McKeever *et al.*, 2005).

Moreover, the rapidity with which a plethora of measures are introduced in the field recalls the philosopher Giorgio Agamben's argument that a 'state of exception' is present as a practice of government. Agamben defines the state of exception as 'a point of imbalance between public law and political fact' that exists at an 'ambiguous, uncertain borderline fringe between the legal and the political'. Commenting on the stuation in Europe up to the present time, he argues that government 'instead of declaring the state of exception prefers to have exceptional laws issued' (Agamben, 2005, p21). This is an important insight with respect to issues relating to asylum seekers and refugees, where a set of political considerations, not least those construed as linked to terrorism and security and media-induced scares regarding the country being 'flooded' by migrants, routinely provoke the implementation of increasingly draconian laws and policies.

It is within this politically charged and unstable environment that asylum claims are made and measures are taken to process them. At the time of writing, the strategies adopted by the British government have resulted in a significant reduction in asylum claims even within a broader European context in which the numbers seeking asylum has reduced. It is interesting to note that the decline in numbers is less notable in France which, in 2005, topped the league of industrialised countries with the most asylum seekers. While the numbers of claims in France are significantly below those reached by the UK and Germany in earlier years, they are relatively high and may be suggestive of the impact of the border control measures taken in the UK (UNHCR, 2007).

For unaccompanied minors seeking to enter the UK, there were a number of distinctive modes of entry with consequences in terms of asylum determination and welfare provision. There were those, described above, who passed through the port in a clandestine manner and, when the opportunity presented itself, left the mode of transport through which entry had been achieved and sought the police to make an asylum claim. Then there were the examples cited above, that include those who spontaneously presented themselves at the port as asylum seekers or those who did so after being detected in the port or its environs. Others entered aiming to unite with contacts in the country and had the intention of entering in an undetected manner, perhaps with the aid of traffickers. These unaccompanied minors, unless apprehended by the authorities, remained invisible, perhaps only coming to the attention of the authorities and the public when some large-scale illegal activity was uncovered.

For those unaccompanied minors who do reach the UK, claims may be made at the point they are intercepted by the authorities typically, in the case of Dover, when they are discovered in the back of a container or when they present themselves to the port authorities and make a claim, or where they make a claim later after having entered the interior of the country. As Derluyn and Broekaert noted in the case of the unaccompanied minors they studied in Belgium, the children usually have very little advice and were often both tired and confused (2005). In ensuring that they have willing and unproblematic customers, smugglers may have talked down the difficulties the unaccompanied minors were likely to experience on arrival in the UK. A member of my research group recalls the following statement by an unaccompanied minor he interviewed:

> They told me after four hours you go into the cities and there is England. You go out and the police they catch you. He told me the police tell you, 'Welcome to England', but for me the police catch me, but they didn't say 'welcome to England'. I didn't know what should happen.

The above quotation reinforces the perception that, while the unaccompanied minors may have a single-minded determination to get to the UK, this may be partially, at least, related to a distorted and conveniently benign view put forward by the smugglers. Here England is not simply the land one enters when the border is crossed, but is identified as consisting of a number of urban areas in which the police, rather than provoking feelings of fear and repression, will respond positively to the unaccompanied minors and actually welcome them. They may thus be advised that rather than plan to avoid the police in England, they should actively seek them out as they offer a route towards safety and security. Here the boy was surprised that the police did not welcome him to the country and at this point experienced disorientation owing to the fact that the narrative presented by the smugglers, on the basis of which he may have sustained himself for the journey, was revealed to be incorrect. This *point of disorientation* in which sustaining narrative was contradicted by stark reality, was something commonly experienced by unaccompanied minors at various stages of their journey and, perhaps most acutely, when they reached their promised land.

On arrival in the UK, many unaccompanied minors describe an experience of getting out of a lorry and wandering around not sure where they are or what to do. Some described not having eaten for up to three or four days, having no money and being unable to speak the language. They could have arrived at any time of day or night and some unaccompanied minors recall walking around a town for hours before seeing the police. The police were an important point of reference in that their presence was a component of the state apparatus that, in its ubiquity, the unaccompanied minors could identify with. By contrast, they normally had little or no conception of the distinctive roles of, for example, immigration officers or social workers. My research student, Chris Endersby, found that in the course of extensive interviewing with unaccompanied minors, while many of the boys he interviewed were surprised by some of the complexities they encountered, they generally took the view that they had been treated well by the authorities. For example, one boy who Endersby refers to as Fari describes the following encounter:

> Then the police came and they took me to the police station and spoke to the interpreter. Then the police said we will take you somewhere else where there is food and you can eat. I was very happy about that. I did not eat for a long time, maybe thirty hours.
>
> (Endersby, 2007)

Having indicated that they were asylum seekers, the unaccompanied minors were normally taken to a police station and then to somewhere where they could receive some food and drink. On the basis of a study in three UK local authority areas, Wade *et al.* report that in cases where an unaccompanied minor is identified at a port of entry, for example Dover, 'referral to a duty social worker at the immigration holding area was normally immediate'. However, in circumstances where they had been identified some time after entry into the country, this contact was likely to be made through people they had met on the streets, siblings or family members or through community organisations (Wade *et al.*, 2005, p40). Despite this, for those identified at the port of entry, the experience of arrival could be deeply disturbing. To take one example from my fieldnotes:

Amir arrived late at night and, as a result of such, was kept waiting at Immigration for a long time before being moved to Dover Detention Centre; a place he recalls as having 'bars on the windows'. He did not submit any details on arrival. The following day he met an Immigration Officer who took his photograph and fingerprints and asked him some questions. Even at this initial interview he said the atmosphere was harsh and he felt as if the officer was pushing him for answers. Following this he was interviewed by social services; regarding his name, date of birth and religion.

(Watters, 2003)

The procedure at the port was that, once identified either though being discovered by the range of scanning and surveillance devices or through approaching officials and claiming asylum, the unaccompanied minor was placed in a holding area of the port, administered by a private security firm. They were subsequently interviewed by immigration officials to determine their identity and route to the UK. In the section below, the reception procedure is examined with specific reference to the pivotal aspect of age assessment.

The politics of reception and age determination

The appropriate reception of asylum seekers and refugees into host societies is a matter of substantial ongoing debate among governmental and non-governmental organisations. Efforts have been made to ensure minimal standards in reception services by issuing policy recommendations and guidelines from a wide range of national and international bodies including the European Commission and the Red Cross (EC, 2003; Red Cross, 2004). As noted, academic contributions have included Foucauldian studies into the rationalities and technologies of immigration control and social support for refugees (Morris, 1998; Ong, 2003; Inda, 2006) and clinically oriented studies into the impact of policies of deterrence on the health and mental health of refugees (Silove *et al.*, 2000; Pourgourides *et al*,. 1996). While the reception and social support of unaccompanied asylum-seeking children is widely recognised as both urgent and highly important, and has been the subject of a range of specific guidelines and recommendations, it has received relatively limited academic investigation.

Internationally, the specific issue of age determination has been recognised as important, as it has a critical role in determining the nature and extent of the social support given to asylum seekers and may have a significant impact on the potential for asylum seekers to be recognised as refugees or be allowed to remain in a country under humanitarian considerations. As in many countries, in the UK the issue is an important one for immigration authorities and local authorities, in that asylum seekers who are classified as over 18 and therefore adults are subject to a range of distinctive policies and practices as compared to those deemed under 18 and therefore 'children'. In this context, children are the responsibility of local authorities and are subject to more extensive programmes of social care, supervision and support than their adult counterparts. While their chances of achieving a successful outcome to their asylum claim is significantly wer than that of adults, most had the benefit of being allowed to remain in the country on humanitarian grounds (Finch, 2005).

The fieldwork on which this section is based was undertaken over a period of six months in 2003, during which time the local authority was actively engaged in reviewing reception procedures for unaccompanied minors and testing a pilot scheme. Here both the established system for receiving unaccompanied minors and the arrangements under the new scheme are examined as both were in existence at the time of the research. As in previous examples, the emphasis is on examining actual practice or 'street level bureaucracy' and revealing the role of laws and policies within this dynamic context. The context is thus broadly one of interrelationship between refugee children and what may loosely be described, following Foucault, as a series of 'specific government apparatuses' (Foucault, 1991, p103). In adopting a Foucauldian approach to these apparatuses, the emphasis is on exploring both the techniques of government and the development of a 'whole complex of savoirs', or forms of knowledge on which these techniques are informed and which are inextricably linked to their development.

The issue of age determination is central to both the determination of the apparatuses of government and the forms of knowledge brought to bear on the asylum seeker. According to the immigration rules applied in the UK, a child is defined as a person under the age of 18 or, in the absence of any documentary evidence, appears to be under that age (Home Office, 2005). Given that a large number of children arrive without the necessary documentation, the matter of age determination assumes central importance. This is apparent at a number of levels. It is central to providing the appropriate legal context for the child to remain in the country. Asylum decisions on children can have, broadly speaking, four potential outcomes; the achievement of refugee status, leave to remain under humanitarian criteria, discretionary leave to remain, or refusal to grant leave to remain. In practice, most separated asylum-seeking children are granted a period of discretionary leave to remain. Figures from the Home Office for 2004 show that out of 3,055 initial decisions, only 2 per cent were recognised as refugees and granted asylum, while three-quarters (72%) were granted a period of discretionary leave. Fourteen per cent were refused any kind of status (Crawley, 2006).

The policy of the UK government in the mid-2000s was not to return unaccompanied asylum-seeking children to their countries of origin unless there were adequate reception and care arrangements in place in those countries. Researchers have been sceptical as to whether a process was undertaken to establish this. According to Finch, 'in practice, no enquiries are usually made about the adequacy of such arrangements, a child is just granted discretionary leave until he or she is eighteen' (Finch, 2005, p58). However, writing in 2006, Crawley argues that the British government is implementing a scheme for the forced return of separated children whose asylum claims have been refused to countries which it considers to be safe (Crawley, 2006, p19). This appeared to be confirmed by a front page headline report in the *Guardian* newspaper in August 2006 which claimed that the Home Office was drawing up plans to 'forcibly repatriate up to 500 children to Vietnam as part of a programme that could see thousands of minors sent back to an uncertain future in the countries where they were born' (*Guardian*, 18th August 2006). In this case, there did appear to have been enquiries undertaken by the government into the reception and care arrangements within the children's home country. UK officials were reported to have investigated the facilities at a state-run orphanage in Vietnam and, finding them inadequate, were considering directly funding care organisations in host countries.

Discretionary leave in the UK was normally granted for a period of three years, or until a child's eighteenth birthday, whichever period was the shortest. The probability of receiving discretionary leave to remain if deemed to be under 18 may be a factor in some adults claiming to be children. Crawley, in a 2006 report for the UK Immigration Law Practitioners Association, argues that in some cases in which age is disputed, the dispute arises because 'an adult claims to be a child because he or she believes this will lead to better treatment or that he or she will be allowed to stay in the UK' (2006, p15). However, she goes on to argue that there are a range of reasons why children, in the sense of being under the age of 18, may appear to be older than they actually are:

> The fact that children have worked and taken on 'adult' responsibilities from an early age, the experiences and traumas associated with migration, differences in cultural norms, and some aspects of physical development, all contribute to the fact that children from other areas of the world may appear older than children brought up in a Western culture and context.
>
> (Ibid., p15)

These points, along with the observation that a third of all births worldwide are not registered, have been made regularly to counter a pervasive culture of disbelief among immigration and welfare institutions in receiving countries, including the UK. In contacts with senior reception and social services staff both in Dover and in a variety of international forums, the general assumption was made that a large number of those presenting to immigration officers as children were in fact adults. This institutional response has also been noted in the US where 'the official assumption is generally that adults will understate their age due to the perceived benefits of being a minor' (Bhabha and Schmidt, 2006, p115).

In the UK the reasons for this presumed deception were viewed by immigration authorities as in accord with Crawley's observation. Being seen as a child generally assured the asylum seeker of the opportunity to stay in the UK until he or she was at least 18 and receive the benefit of a range of welfare provisions. Most immediately, it had considerable practical consequences for the various agencies involved in the care of asylum seekers. If an asylum seeker was assessed as being under 18, he or she was placed in local authority control that was responsible for undertaking a comprehensive assessment of the child's needs and providing a range of assistance including supported accommodation, a care plan and placement in a school or college. The local authority initially provided the funding for this care although it would claim a reimbursement for these expenses from central government.

Age determination was also significant for the asylum seekers themselves in that it has a great impact on the quality of their experience in the UK. Those who were judged to be under the age of 18 were normally placed in local residential centres or, in some cases, foster care, while adult asylum seekers were placed under the care of the Home Office National Asylum Support Service (NASS). The latter were sometimes placed in detention or in emergency accommodation before being 'dispersed' to areas of the UK away from the economically affluent and densely populated south east. Unaccompanied children were not normally the subjects of detention although between 1994 and 2001 a small proportion of children were reported to be in detention (Ayotte and Williamson, 2001). The figure is quite different for children in families with Crawley reporting that every year approximately 2,000 children are detained in the UK with a significant negative impact on child welfare (ibid., p41).

Physiologically based processes of age determination are both complex and controversial. According to guidelines issued by the Royal College of Paediatrics and Child Health in 1999, 'Age determination is an inexact science and the margin of error can sometimes be as much as 5 years on either side' (1999). This view is echoed in the comments of senior clinicians in the US. Bhabha and Schmidt report the following comment from a prominent doctor involved in the process,

> I am extremely troubled by the inaccuracy of the current INS practice of using bone age and dental age standards to judge chronological age among undocumented immigrants and asylum seekers...chronologic age, dental age and skeletal age are not necessarily the same in a given individual. In fact, deviation among these three 'ages' is common and well appreciated in paediatric, medical and dental practice. Discrepancies among these ages can amount to as much as five years.
>
> (Bhabha and Schmidt, 2006, p117)

In the Netherlands doctors have refused to undertake X-rays aimed at determining age and the state contracts in Belgian doctors to do this work (Essakkili, 2007). Bhabha and Schmidt report that procedures such as wrist and dental procedures have been completely discarded in the UK in favour of a more holistic assessment.

The inexactitude of the process is of critical importance in a context in which the assessed age of a high proportion of unaccompanied minors entering industrialised countries is between 15 and 18 years old. In a recent judicial review, the unreliability of anthropomorphic measurement was highlighted and the potential for accurate age determination was noted to be further eroded in instances where the individual is from a different ethnic and cultural background.[3] In the absence of reliable anthropomorphic methods, local authorities in the UK were recommended to adopt a range of methods for assessing age including physical appearance and demeanour, manner of interaction with the assessing worker, social history and developmental considerations. It has also been noted that 'life experience and trauma may impact on the aging process' (London boroughs of Hillingdon and Croydon, 2004). Recent practice guidelines also draw attention to the contexts in which young asylum seekers are interviewed and the potential impact of the environment on age assessment.

> It is very important to ensure that the young person understands the role of the assessing worker, and comprehends the interpreter. Attention should also be paid to the level of tiredness, trauma, bewilderment and anxiety that may be present for the young person. The ethnicity, culture, and customs of the person being assessed must be a key focus throughout the assessment.
>
> (London boroughs of Hillingdon and Croydon, 2004)

Against this background, the formal position of the Home Office was that in instances where the individuals' appearance strongly suggests an age of over 18 years, they should be treated as such (Home Office, 2000). However, in borderline cases the Immigration Service will continue to 'give the applicant the benefit of the doubt and deal with the applicant as a minor'. The Immigration Service will then refer the applicant to the local authority for support under the Children Act 1989. It will then conduct an assessment and, on the basis of this, may refer the individual back to the Immigration Service and, on the basis of the assessment, the Immigration Service will treat the individual as an adult unless they can prove otherwise.

These policies introduce a complex interrelationship between two principal agencies involved in the management and care of asylum seekers, who sit at the intersection of distinctive administrative processes. An initial assessment of age is typically undertaken by immigration officials at a port of entry and based on the documentary and verbal evidence given by asylum seekers and a visual inspection by an immigration officer. Where there is an element of doubt, the matter was referred to a chief immigration officer who determined whether the asylum seeker is clearly over 18. In these instances, the individual was referred to the National Asylum Support Service to undertake an assessment of social care needs and arrange for the asylum seeker to be placed in emergency accommodation or detention. As noted above, borderline cases were given the 'benefit of the doubt' by immigration officials and sent to the local authority social service department for care under the Children Act 1989.

Immigration officials are not required to be specialists in any of the areas relating to age assessment and their approach is largely informed by 'common sense' and their collective experience in the job. This is not to disparage their role in the process, but to highlight the potential discrepancies that exist in terms of 'expert knowledge' between these agencies. Social service departments are the principal statutory agency responsible for child welfare and, as such, have a correspondingly large resource of professional knowledge and expertise in the field. Once the 'borderline' asylum seeker was referred to social services, this expertise could be mobilised in undertaking a more wide-ranging assessment drawing on the range of contextual, social and developmental factors referred to above. This professional expertise would be deferred to even if it contradicted the initial assessment of the immigration service.

Given the components of age assessments outlined above, an early assessment following arrival at a port of entry appeared inappropriate. The young person is likely to have arrived feeling very tired and disoriented. He or she may have had a physically and emotionally arduous journey huddled in the back of a container lorry, cargo ship or other form of transport and was likely to feel very anxious about reception in the host country and have a minimal knowledge of the language and country. These feelings may be compounded by the impact of highly stressful events in the country of origin and in flight (Silove *et al.*, 2000). The local authority that was the subject of this study took these factors into account in proposing a new system for receiving unaccompanied asylum-seeking children. This system is examined below and the implications of this new approach are assessed. Before doing so it is appropriate to provide some broader contextual information about the port of entry and young unaccompanied asylum seekers arriving in the UK.

As numbers of asylum seekers entering the UK increased dramatically during the 1990s and early 2000s, the port of Dover became a major site for the reception and initial processing of asylum applicants. To cope with increasing numbers the amount of immigration officers and police at the port increased and a range of voluntary and private sector organisations were contracted to support statutory services. A small voluntary organisation, Migrant Helpline, based at the port received a contract from the Home Office to expand its activities to include assessment of the social care needs of adult asylum seekers. Following assessment, Migrant Helpline would find the applicant temporary accommodation while the asylum application was being considered. Besides the agencies dealing with the arrival of asylum seekers, the Home Office introduced an Immigration Removal Centre in 2002 run by the Prisons Service. The building was originally a fort built in Napoleonic times, complete with moat and contains residential space for 316 detainees. Following an inspection of the Centre undertaken in 2004 by Her Majesty's Chief Inspector of Prisons, the Chief Inspector commented in her report on the 'forbidding appearance' of the Centre, mitigated to some degree by the attempts of staff to offer a regime that differentiated detainees from prisoners (Her Majesty's Chief Inspector of Prisons, 2004). Between 2000 and 2003, the port of Dover police estimate that 5,181 illegal entrants were arrested and detained while trying to enter the UK from continental Europe (port of Dover police, 2003). Besides those seeking to enter clandestinely, there were those who claimed asylum at the port of entry.

In line with national statistics, Kent County Council (the local authority that covered Dover and surrounding areas) statistics incorporating the port of Dover, showed approximately 80 to 100 unaccompanied minors being referred to social services each month between 2002 and 2003. At the end of 2003, Kent County Council was supporting 1,200 unaccompanied minors, the majority of whom were male and aged between 16 and 17. From 2003 a further significant consideration was whether the unaccompanied minor was under or over 16. If deemed under 16, the child was usually supported under section 20 of the Children Act 1989. This support required a regularly reviewed care plan, placement in foster or residential care and placement within a school or college within 20 days taken into care by social services. By contrast, those deemed over 16 wei to a less intensive, and less expensive, regime of care under section 17 (that included placement in independent or semi-independent accommodation ana some financial support. The importance of this distinction was reinforced by policy decisions taken by the Home Office, which allowed for a significantly higher rate of reimbursement for the expenses incurred by local authorities for children under 16 (Liddicott, 2003).

The economic rationality underpinning these measures manifested in concrete terms in the trajectories followed by unaccompanied minors after arrival. Following arrival, they were subjected to a range of mechanisms of surveillance including examination of documents, photographing and fingerprinting. They had a 'screening interview' with immigration officers that included eliciting biographical data and evidence of the route taken to enter the country. This was a critical juncture for the unaccompanied minor, as it was the context in which a judgement is made about age. If the unaccompanied minor was judged to be over 18 he or she was treated as an adult and normally directed either towards an assessment by Migrant Helpline or, if the claim is deemed manifestly unfounded, detention. Those judged to be between 16 and 17 were referred to Finding Your Feet, a project commissioned by the local authority. This agency undertook an assessment of needs and placed the unaccompanied minor in a residential home where they experienced a degree of independent living. As noted above, those deemed to be under 16 were placed in residential care. It should be added that this option was not available in the case of the relatively small number of unaccompanied asylum-seeking girls who were routinely placed in foster care. For those seeking asylum at the port the following diagram is illustrative of the complexities of the bureaucratic processes operating within the UK in 2004 (see Figure 4.1).

It is notable that within hours a screening interview was undertaken and a judgement of the age of the unaccompanied minors was made on the basis of this and of:

- documentation and/or statements presented by the unaccompanied minors
- visual inspection by an immigration officer
- where there was doubt, the judgement of a Chief Immigration Officer as to whether the unaccompanied minor was 'clearly over 18'.

The conditions at the initial screening interview were typically highly unfavourable to an objective assessment of age. The unaccompanied minors were often tired, fearful and confused, with no independent advice about the asylum process and perhaps schooled in what to say by interested adults. What was said at the initial screening formed part of the asylum determination process and disparities between what was initially presented and evidence given later could form a basis for the rejection of an asylum claim.

Thus unaccompanied asylum-seeking children were categorised and placed in distinctive regimes of care and control depending on age assessment and gender.

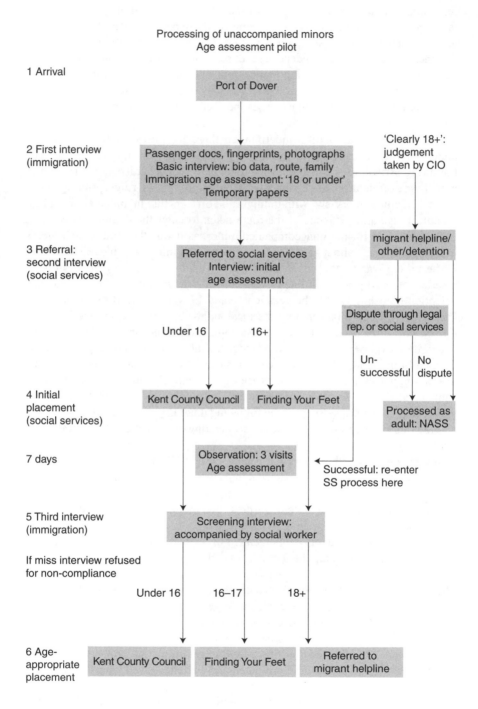

Processing of unaccompanied minors
Age assessment pilot

1 Arrival

Port of Dover

2 First interview
(immigration)

Passenger docs, fingerprints, photographs
Basic interview: bio data, route, family
Immigration age assessment: '18 or under'
Temporary papers

'Clearly 18+':
judgement
taken by CIO

3 Referral:
second interview
(social services)

Referred to social services
Interview: initial
age assessment

migrant helpline/
other/detention

Under 16   16+

Dispute through legal
rep. or social services

Un-   No
successful dispute

4 Initial
placement
(social services)

Kent County Council   Finding Your Feet

Processed as
adult: NASS

7 days

Observation: 3 visits
Age assessment

Successful: re-enter
SS process here

5 Third interview
(immigration)

Screening interview:
accompanied by social worker

If miss interview refused
for non-compliance

Under 16   16–17   18+

6 Age-
appropriate
placement

Kent County Council   Finding Your Feet

Referred to
migrant helpline

Figure 4.1 Port of entry procedures – Dover

It is interesting to consider the development and operation of these regimes from a Foucauldian governmentality perspective. Morris has fruitfully adopted such an approach in her detailed analysis of the development of immigration controls in the UK by Conservative administrations in the 1980s and 1990s. She noted a gradual convergence between mechanisms of immigration control and social welfare provisions within the UK (Morris, 1998). She concludes her analysis by commenting that, while a governmentality approach can be enlightening in the examination of the rationality and techniques for managing immigration, it has limitations as it does not account for processes through which individuals may fall outside of government control. She comments that:

> While resource constraints and the policy of deterrence mean strict eligibility, this creates a population of people present on the territory but outside of all provision. Ironically, this denial of rights also means there is no mechanism for policing this group; destitute and inadequately documented, they are not readily traceable.
>
> (Morris, 1998, p969)

It is notable that some of the gaps that Morris documents as giving rise to this phenomenon have been addressed by an extension of the mechanisms of control through the development of the National Asylum Support Service (NASS), an agency of the Home Office that combines surveillance and control of asylum seekers with the administration of social provisions. NASS effectively fills previous gaps between central and local government by removing the obligation of local authorities to directly provide housing for adult asylum seekers. However, it is arguable that in seeking to provide a tough and seamless system of immigration control and social provision, many would-be asylum seekers were excluding themselves from the process by entering the country clandestinely and seeking to survive without making an asylum application. As noted above, issues concerning the interface between local and national government remain salient with respect to asylum-seeking children and the fissures relating to service provision highlighted by Morris remain problematic for this group. The issue of age determination is a case in point and one that represents acutely the complexities of the interface between the Immigration Authority and local government within a specific geographical locality.

The introduction of a pilot scheme to improve reception arrangements for unaccompanied minors can be examined within this context of an expansion of the rationality and techniques of governmentality to this group. The scheme sought to address real and potential fissures in the operation of reception arrangements and age determination. It operated for four months between February and May 2003. Under the scheme, the responsibility for establishing the unaccompanied minor's date of birth was transferred from the Immigration Authorities to the local authority Social Services Department (SSD). To achieve this, the interview conducted by the Immigration Authority (IA) was split into two stages. The first was to be viewed as a basic interview conducted by the IA shortly after the unaccompanied minor's arrival in the UK. This was aimed at obtaining information about the route of entry into the UK, his or her family and biographical details. The unaccompanied minors would be fingerprinted and photographed and those judged by the Chief Immigration Officer to be mani-festly over 18 would be transferred to adult services as before. Those who remained were issued with temporary papers and released into the care of the SSD for seven days. Social services would, during this period, attempt to build trust and a rapport with the unaccompanied minors and use their experience to arrive at an appropriate age assessment. An outcome of this assessment was the production of a date of birth agreed between the two agencies.

A central objective of the pilot was, therefore, to develop an agreed approach towards age assessment that drew on the expertise of social services and which would minimise the potential for subsequent age disputes. Besides administrative and operational considerations, it was also hoped that the pilot would result in more generally cohesive working arrangements between the IA and SSD. It also had an explicitly humanitarian aspect in that emphasis was placed on giving the unaccompanied minors time to rest and calm down after an arduous journey in the hope that these more favourable circumstances would lead to a more accurate understanding of their needs and circumstances.

For practical operational reasons, the pilot study was only applied to those asy-lum seekers presenting themselves as seeking asylum at the port of entry. Those who entered the country clandestinely and were typically found in the back of lor-ries in the port were subject to the established system. Over the period of four months, 39 unaccompanied minors were included in the pilot and 150 who entered clandestinely were processed in the usual way. Besides their mode of entry, further distinguishing features of the two groups were subsequently identi-fied. Of the pilot group, 72 per cent were male and 28 per cent female, while all of the 150 people who entered clandestinely were male. The overwhelming majority of both groups were in the 16 to 18 age range but, interestingly, a few who entered clandestinely were very young children aged between 7 and 11 years old. It is inappropriate of course to draw conclusions from such small samples. The higher numbers of girls applying for asylum at the port of entry and the pres-ence of relatively young children arriving clandestinely, does however, suggest topics for further investigation not least to ascertain the personal circumstances that led these children to arrive at the port in these ways.

A comparative analysis of the process undergone by the two groups involved in the study indicated that there were much more rigorous measures taken with respect to the pilot group. For this entire group, a date of birth was established by social services and this formed a basis for their asylum application. Ten of those assessed under the pilot scheme were given an age different from the one they gave to the immigration authorities. Nine were assessed as being older and only one assessed as being younger. In general, service providers from both social ser-vices and immigration expressed satisfaction with the operation of the pilot scheme as it improved interagency co-operation and brought practice more into line with international conventions and guidelines.

However, three significant problem areas remained. Although the researchers were only able to interview a small number of unaccompanied minors included in the sample, they gave an impression of participating in a process that they did not understand, some aspects of which they experienced as hostile. The process often involved multiple moves to different forms of accommodation, and meetings with personnel from a variety of agencies. Secondly, the role of social services in the final screening interview was unclear. One unaccompanied minor said he was accompanied by two social workers to his final screening interview, neither said a word and their presence was not helpful to him in any way. A third significant feature was the high level of absconding amongst both groups, and was significantly higher among the pilot group. On the basis of an examination of the files of 34 children involved in the pilot study and 62 involved in the regular procedure, 17 per cent of the pilot group and 8 per cent of the regular group absconded. Absconding had potentially dire consequences for the pilot group as they had removed themselves from services prior to receiving the forms available at the screening interview necessary to process their asylum application. They thus form a group identified by Morris (1998) as 'present in the territory but outside of all provision', albeit in this instance from a later decade and from within differing administrative and policy contexts. A difference between rates of absconding between the mainstream service and the pilot may be that the former discouraged absconding and mitigated some of its potential ill effects by having a swifter throughput including the rapid issuing of Asylum Registration Cards.

The study of age-assessment procedures has implications for the development of policies and practices towards unaccompanied minors at ports of entry and for the development of further academic research. In terms of policy and practice, the outcome of age assessment was, as noted, of critical importance to the regime of care experienced by the asylum seekers. It also determined the agencies that would deliver care and the legal context in which it would be provided. Once the asylum seeker falls, at the age of 18, outside of the regime of childcare under the Children Act, he or she then becomes the responsibility of the Home Office and could, in circumstances where an asylum claim had been unsuccessful, be subject to deportation. While the pilot scheme described here was too limited in scope to have a dramatic impact on the process of reception and age determination, it nevertheless provided evidence of a potentially more efficient and humane mechanism. It improved interagency understanding and co-operation, and provided a welcome breathing space for unaccompanied minors before their main screening interview. As noted, it also served to bring the process closer in line with national and international conventions and guidelines (Bhabha and Finch, 2006).

Refugee children and the mixed economy of care

Besides the major demarcation between the treatment of children and adults, there was a clear operational distinction between the referral process and the care regimes of those deemed to be under and over 16. The latter were referred to an organisation called Finding Your Feet, a section of a large local independent service provider, Kent Community Housing Trust, with, in the mid-2000s, approximately 1,500 staff , a regular turnover of £25 million and £13 million in assets. It established a project with funding from the local authority, Kent County Council, to provide temporary accommodation for 25 unaccompanied minors while more long-term accommodation was found. This position changed in response to increases in numbers and in the early 2000s Finding Your Feet became responsible for offering accommodation to significant numbers of unaccompanied minors entering Kent through the establishment of a major reception centre and outreach programmes. As will be explored in more detail below, the regime of care under which these older children were placed allowed for a relatively low level of support that could be provided by low paid staff without social work qualifications.

This 'contracting out' of care followed a broader approach, the origins of which can be found in the welfare reforms of the government of Margaret Thatcher in the mid-1980s. These were underpinned by an ideological commitment to bring a culture of the marketplace into health and social care, resulting in a range of legislative changes, the impact of which began to be felt acutely in the 1990s (Bartlett *et al.*, 1998). Kent Community Housing Trust, which was established in 1990, was representative of a wider shift in social care from direct service provision to the purchasing of services by government bodies. The potential providers included a range of voluntary and private organisations that would negotiate the best value for money contracts with the purchaser.

The legislative framework for the care and protection of children in the UK is provided by the Children Act 1989. Part 3 of the Act provides the legal framework for local authority support for children and families. Two sections in particular are highly relevant to the local authority response to unaccompanied minors. Section 17 stipulates a general duty of every local authority to 'safeguard and promote the welfare of children within their area who are in need'. Further, 'every local authority shall facilitate the provision by others (including in particular voluntary organisations) of services which the authority have power to provide' and 'may make such arrangements as they see fit for any person to act on their behalf in the provision of any such service'.

As such, this section may be characterised as providing a directive that allows local authorities to provide care at 'arm's length' through contracting out services from voluntary and private organisations. The author of a recent report observes that, with respect to UASC, local authorities have commonly used Section 17 to provide unaccompanied children with financial support and accommodation ranging from supported lodgings to a B&B, a privately rented shared house or a hostel (Free, 2005). Wade and colleagues have pointed to the wide disparities in the quality of services provided under Section 17:

> At one extreme, rudimentary assessments led to placements in unsupported shared housing that provided limited (if any) social work contact and support. Placement and support arrangements were routine and resource led.

At the other extreme, where support was provided by children's teams or, to a lesser extent, by dedicated support agencies, the overall package of support for young people was largely indistinguishable from that provided to looked after children.

(Wade *et al.*, 2005, p3)

By contrast, Section 20 of the Act provides a context in which children are 'looked after' by the local authority. The criteria for being looked after under Section 20 includes the following:

- there being no person who has parental responsibility for him *(sic)*
- his being lost or abandoned
- the person who has been caring for him being prevented (whether or not permanently, and for whatever reason) from providing him with suitable accommodation and/or care.

(HMSO, 1989)

Children under Section 20 are 'looked after' and have traditionally been placed in a foster or residential home. They receive the support of an allocated social worker, have a care plan and regular statutory reviews, receive financial support and are entitled to full 'leaving care' services, the latter involving 'a pathway plan and a personal advisor to co-ordinate a support package through to the age of 21, or beyond if continuing in education' (Wade *et al.*, 2005, p185).

A series of Court of Appeal judgements cast doubt on local authorities' powers to help families and children with accommodation under Section 17 of the Act and it was amended in 2002. The amendment clarified the position to the effect that local authorities' functions under Section 17 may include 'providing accommodation, giving assistance in kind or, in exceptional circumstances, in cash'. However, a local authority circular issued in 2003 stipulated that 'the power to provide accommodation under section 17 will almost always concern children needing to be accommodated with their families' (Department of Health, 2003). A child accommodated under this section of the Act would not be considered 'looked after' and would not benefit from the provisions of the Children (Leaving Care) Act 2000.

The circular added that the local authority should undertake an assessment based on statutory guidance set out in the Framework for the Assessment of Children in Need and their Families and then use the findings of this assessment to determine whether the child should be accommodated under Section 20 of the Children Act or supported by other services under Section 17. A highly relevant passage from the circular comments specifically on the position of unaccompanied minors to the effect that,

where a child has no parent or guardian in this country, perhaps because he has arrived alone seeking asylum, the presumption should be that he would fall within the scope of Section 20 and become looked after, unless the needs assessment reveals particular factors which would suggest that an alternative response would be more appropriate.

(Department of Health, 2003)

A further legislative development had policy implications here. The Hillingdon judgement refers to the result of a judicial review taken out in relation to the London borough of Hillingdon. It concluded that some former unaccompanied minors who had been 'assisted' under Section 17 of the Act had essentially been 'looked after' as defined by Section 20 and were therefore entitled to leaving care support. As stated in a recent report, 'The judgement established in law that Section 17 of the Children Act 1989 should not routinely be used to meet the accommodation and support needs of unaccompanied children' (Free, 2005). The implications for local authorities have been summarised as follows:

- All unaccompanied children should, on arrival, be supported under Section 20 of the Children Act until an assessment is carried out.
- Based on an assessment of need, most unaccompanied children should be provided with Section 20 support including 16–17 year olds.
- The majority of unaccompanied young people will be entitled to leaving care services.
- Section 17 can be used to accommodate unaccompanied children in exceptional circumstances.

(Free, 2005, p12)

A recent survey, undertaken by Save the Children, of 18 local authorities indicated a mixed picture of the use of Section 20 support for unaccompanied asylum-seeking children (Free, 2005). Twelve of the local authorities surveyed were providing Section 20 support for all unaccompanied minors. Three were providing a form of 'enhanced' Section 17 support and were planning to gradually move to Section 20 support. Three offered Section 17 support and had no plans for changing this. The key findings of the survey included: variation in the quality and provision of leaving care services, concerns among local authority staff about the quality and level of support they were able to provide, the specific problems encountered in trying to provide services to unaccompanied minors who were at the 'end of the line' in that they had exhausted all legal avenues for staying in the country and were faced with deportation. Further reported concerns included the perceived inadequacy of grants from the Home Office and problems in their administration, the difficulty in gaining support for work with unaccompanied minors from other agencies, negative attitudes of staff to asylum seekers and a lack of senior management and local counsellor support for work in this area.

These findings point again to the complex legal and policy interfaces in which unaccompanied asylum-seeking children are located. On the one hand, the Home Office and, specifically, immigration services are concerned with the security of national borders and the monitoring and control of would-be immigrants pending the determination of legal status. On the other, local authorities have the statutory responsibility for the care of unaccompanied minors under legislation aimed at enhancing the standards of care for children in need, in accordance with international conventions and national and international research and guidelines on good practice. These distinctive areas of concern gave rise to potentially competing agendas and disagreement over the appropriate allocation of resources.

The economic competitiveness of would-be providers was enhanced by the employment of low paid staff with minimal qualifications to undertake a range of social care tasks. The service for unaccompanied minors was no exception and offered an opportunity to minimise costs. This process was crucially supported by the fact that some categories of children who were deemed less vulnerable could be cared for under Section 17 of the Children Act in which there was a lower requirement for the interventions of qualified social work staff. In Kent, to meet the expanding numbers of unaccompanied minors aged between 16 and 17, the contract with the housing trust increased in size and scope and included the opening of a new residential facility. These developments were also influenced by the financial rules and regulations governing the relationship between central and local government whereby local government could claim a standard annually adjusted refund for each unaccompanied minor that it looked after. The Home Office determined the level of grant based on age, with 16- and 17-year-olds getting half of the level of grant of under-16s. This suggested radically different criteria to that offered by local authorities who would normally view the level of grant as appropriately determined by the level of need. Clearly, where Section 20 care was provided, this was unlikely to require a significantly lower level of input for a 17-year-old than a 15- or 16-year-old.

The funding mechanisms were thus established whereby a higher level of payment was available for those who first applied for asylum before the age of 16 and those aged between 16 and 17. As Wade *et al.* have observed, studies have pointed to this distinction as being an 'important driver of differentiated services for unaccompanied young people' (Wade *et al.*, 2005, p8). Local government representatives reported receiving conflicting messages from different departments of central government about the extent to which the provision for children should be based on need and not age. Acute problems emerged such as the situation of those who had been placed in foster care when under 16 and for whom it was difficult to sustain the placement after the child's sixteenth birthday owing to a lack of funds (Free, 2005, p33). Moreover a widespread perception existed among local authorities that the level of payment was insufficient to meet the cost of provision. Free reported that 'local authority departments said they were running on a deficit. The Home Office has stated that the grant is to *help* local authorities provide support to unaccompanied young people and was never intended to cover all the costs' (ibid., p34).

Against this background, at the time of writing measures are being taken by central government to change the role of social work teams at ports of entry to work as adjuncts to immigration services, thus reducing the gap between the immigration and welfare trajectories. There is a clear financial rationality behind these proposals. In 2005, the 6,000 unaccompanied asylum-seeking children supported by local authorities comprised less than 10 per cent of cases, but consumed roughly 25 per cent of the Home Office budget. New proposals set social work teams targets in respect of turning away age disputed clients, reducing repeated age assessment, and assessing more clients claiming to be 15 or less as actually being aged between 16 and 17. The proposals are expected to bring in savings of £1.5 million over a three-year period. The unpublished project proposal ironically comments on the unpredictability of flows of refugee children and the inextricable linkage to international events such as those affecting Afghanistan and Iraq while, simultaneously, being pervaded by a culture of disbelief concerning the veracity of asylum claims and statements of age.

'Safe Case Transfer'

The arrival of significant numbers of unaccompanied asylum-seeking children through the port of Dover thus presented very significant challenges to social care, health and education providers in the south east. Within the legislative framework in which children were placed, social services had a pivotal role in the assessment of needs and in the co-ordination of care. For those children who were 'looked after' under Section 20 of the Children Act 1989, this often included placement with a foster carer or in a residential home with the support of an allocated social worker and, if over 16, a personal advisor, a care or pathway plan and financial support (Crawley, 2006, p22). Those who were 'looked after' also had eligibility for 'leaving care services' up to the age of 21, and beyond if they continued in education. As Wade *et al.* have noted, unaccompanied minors were eligible for these services 'at least to the point where they receive a final negative adjudication on their asylum claims and fail to comply with removal directions'. The services included requirements to prepare young people for adult life, to assess and to meet their needs and to provide pathway plans and personal advisors (Wade *et al.*, 2005, p8). As noted above, those under Section 17 had a much more circumscribed regime of care, which was routinely terminated when the young person reached the age of 18 (ibid.).

Faced with increasing numbers of unaccompanied minors claiming asylum in the UK in the early to mid-2000s, local authorities adopted two basic strategies; either to manage the situation by developing cost-effective measures within the local authority area or to seek contracts for 'out of county' placements. This latter approach was consistent with the broader strategy towards adult asylum seekers who were routinely offered packages of support only if they agreed to move to allocated addresses outside of the densely populated and highly expensive south east of England. Thus the National Asylum Support Service established by the Home Office negotiated contracts with local authorities in the Midlands, the north of England and Scotland to receive asylum seekers and accommodate them in underused properties typically managed by a range of private providers. The idea of dispersal outside of the south east usually came as a considerable shock to asylum seekers whose aspirations were typically linked to an idea of living in

London or its environs. Often they had no knowledge of England beyond what they have heard of London and knew it as a place with the potential to find work and where there may be social networks of people from the same geographical regions, possibly including kin.

Besides these more positive associations, there was concern that, if moved to other parts of the UK, they may be subjected to abuse or even physical attack. One young Iranian asylum seeker interviewed at the Refugee Council in London reported that a friend of his had been subjected to a racial attack in Dover. After claiming asylum he was dispersed to a northern English town where he described himself as being very bored and isolated. The street he was sent to was a centre for drug dealers and he expressed anger at the Home Office for sending him to this environment. He and a friend of his experienced a racial attack and, after being subsequently moved to another location, he reported being attacked again. These incidences exacerbated mental health problems he had initially experienced in Iran and, as a consequence of his condition, he was moved back to London where he received treatment at a psychiatric hospital. He made the following comment about the experience of dispersal outside of London;

> Why send me to this place, send me to a big city. I'm OK in London, it's multi-ethnic and I feel safe. You have visibility in a small town and you feel unsafe. Also, I need to maintain links with my home country and it is possible to do that in London.
>
> (Watters, 2002a, p13)

Asylum seekers often expressed a deep concern with the possible deleterious effects of being moved outside of the capital or the south east. The comment about 'visibility' was representative of a widespread view, often expressed in similar terms in interviews and reported by staff working with asylum seekers. The sheer size and diversity of the multi-ethnic populations of London were felt to be a protection against possible hostility from elements in the host society. Asylum seekers had heard reports of people being sent to impoverished and violent housing estates where they stood out as virtually the only people with a different skin colour. The potential for hostility was exacerbated further by widespread perceptions generated by sections of the media that asylum seekers were cynical and unscrupulous manipulators of the British welfare system. Since the 9/11 attacks on New York and subsequent attacks and attempted attacks in the UK, asylum seekers of North-African appearance felt particularly vulnerable as public sensibilities increasingly distinguished them as outsiders and not part of the UK's settled minority ethnic population which was seen as primarily of South Asian or Afro-Caribbean descent.

Despite these concerns, economic rationality dictated the expansion of a policy of dispersal and it became a central modus operandi of the asylum system. The placement of each asylum seeker outside of the south east was thus achieved as the result of a complex web of financial arrangements; between the Home Office and local government and between local government and a range of 'service providers' from the private and voluntary sectors. A number of private service providers made considerable profits from these arrangements while delivering services that were far below the required standards. It is not possible to review the overall impact of dispersal here but a few salient aspects may be identified. One feature was that local communities often felt that asylum seekers were simply thrust upon them without consultation and that they received more favourable accommodation and services than locals. They were often placed in run-down areas where the general standards of accommodation were low and where there was already local disquiet about the standard of services. On visiting one housing estate in Glasgow where asylum seekers had been placed in a tower block, locals complained that they had seen the council go in to 'do repairs and deliver new televisions and washing machines' when locals had been 'waiting for months to have damp treated' (Watters, 2001c). Local resentment in areas of dispersal often grew from existing prejudice but was sometimes stoked by insensitive policies and practices of receiving authorities, including an absence of preliminary consultation with communities. They were also routinely stoked by predominantly hostile media coverage. There were a number of instances in which the policy had tragic human consequences, for example, in the murder of a young Kurdish asylum seeker in Glasgow and numerous violent assaults in dispersal areas.

In contrast to this bleak picture, dispersal did result in a number of more positive outcomes for both asylum seekers and local communities. Local charitable community organisations frequently welcomed the arrival of the asylum seekers and developed a wide range of supportive services for example in the fields of counselling, advocacy, the arts and sports. There was a growth and expansion in the already extensive number of refugee community organisations (Audit Commission, 2000). Key support organisations, for example, the London-based Medical Foundation for the Care of Victims of Torture, developed their capacity in dispersal areas, resulting in the establishment of a permanent centre in Manchester. Such was the level of good will in some areas that voluntary sector initiatives failed, not because of a lack of volunteers but because of insufficient numbers of asylum seekers to take up the services. As Kristal Logghe has observed from a study of community responses to asylum seekers in the Netherlands, the relationship between volunteers and the asylum seekers they try to help is often complex, with the former holding sometimes idealised visions of what asylum seekers will be like and then experiencing disillusionment when they fail to meet expectations (personal communication).

Against this chequered background, local authorities in the south east sought to address the financial constraints arising from the introduction of significant numbers of unaccompanied minors by sending them 'out of county' into the care of another local authority. Kent County Council had routinely placed significant numbers of minors outside the county including a total of 200 sent to Manchester in 2004. Placement of this kind was quite commonplace, with evidence that this procedure was undertaken for around two-fifths of all unaccompanied minors, despite evidence that social workers faced specific challenges in supporting unaccompanied minors in this way and the children had specific difficulties in accessing the required services. Wade and his colleagues noted problems in accessing key workers and social workers and concluded that 'the provision of consistent support to young people placed out of authority was often more difficult to achieve' (Wade *et al.*, 2005, p79). The limitations of these types of placement were increasingly recognised by agencies responsible for the monitoring of social work services and by local authorities themselves. Furthermore, a combination of issues relating to the care of asylum-seeking unaccompanied minors presented local authorities with serious challenges.

Firstly, there was, following the Hillingdon Judgement, an increasing emphasis on the necessity to place unaccompanied minors in the category of 'looked after' under Section 20. This challenged local authorities to provide a wider range of intensive professionalised services to this group and diminished their ability to contract out aspects of care to relatively low cost third parties. A further and related aspect was the requirement to provide an integrated and comprehensive range of services drawing on interagency collaboration with key providers of health, education and housing services. Further, there was extension of the category 'looked after' to those aged between 16 and 17 and consequent demand to continue to provide 'leaving care' services while the young person was in education, possibly until the age of 21. Finally, there was the overarching problem of increasingly acute financial pressures deriving from the perceived inadequacy of the Home Office grant.

To seek to address these problems Kent County Council developed the idea of 'Safe Case Transfer' whereby unaccompanied minors who had usually arrived through Dover and were the responsibility of the local authority, would be transferred out of the county but in a manner that was consistent with the principles of care underpinning Section 20. The Strategic Director of Social Services wrote to potentially interested parties in 2002 to explore the possibility of partnerships to develop a new model of care and, after a long process of negotiation, the Association of Greater Manchester Authorities was selected to develop a pilot programme. While the pilot was to involve a relatively modest number of 30 unaccompanied minors, it was developed through an extensive process of consultation and negotiation spanning a period of three years. It included a Project Board, an Operational Working Party, a Financial Working Party and a Policy Officer as well as a publicity strategy involving all of the press officers of the participating authorities. A project steering group consisting of 13 agencies collaborated to produce an extensive 'Safe Case Transfer Policies and Procedures Manual'. This included a set of meticulously formulated procedures covering a wide range of aspects of the children's care including assessment by social work staff, physical transfer, procedures for age assessment, access to legal advice and advocacy, the standard of accommodation offered and access to education, health care, leisure and social activities. The services offered to the unaccompanied minors were also informed by consultation with them through focus groups. On the basis of one such group run in 2004 prior to the implementation of the project, the unaccompanied minors made the following requests of social services: access to interpreters, decent housing, an identified key worker who would help them with legal, health and housing issues and a responsible adult who would oversee all aspects of their care. The various bodies established to implement the project incorporated these aspects into the planning process.

The core idea behind the Safe Case Transfer project was that it would offer a 'prototype' for the broader development of social care services for unaccompanied minors across the UK. It had the potential to meet both the emerging more stringent requirements of Section 20 care for unaccompanied minors between 16 and 18 and simultaneously avoid the economic pressures associated with providing care within the south east of England. In practical terms it had proved to be extremely challenging for social services to offer an integrated programme of care from residential establishments located often in rural or semi-rural locations. The shift to a northern metropolitan area offered the opportunity to develop a network of services within easy travelling distance. It was also viewed as being more appropriate because the Manchester area was highly ethnically diverse and was viewed by the participating authorities as offering access to cultures that were closer to those of the unaccompanied minors.

The initial pilot project was designed for 30 male unaccompanied minors aged between 16 and 17 of Afghan or Kurdish background. Additional criteria were that the boys had no significant health problems and no family ties in the south east. The project was externally evaluated and the lessons arising from it were designed to inform the development of a wider range of services based on the principles of safe case transfer. The 30 unaccompanied minors who took part in the project were recruited from a residential centre for unaccompanied minors in Kent. The centre had been opened in 1999 on the site of an existing youth and community service for children who were in the care of the Social Services Department. It was established as a reception and assessment centre and as such represented an acknowledgement that the unaccompanied minors entering Kent were vulnerable and in need of specialist care and protection (Endersby, 2007). In interviews with staff at the centre, undertaken by the author in late 2005, changes affecting the service from January 2005 were described as pivotal in the development of the Safe Case Transfer project. Until then the centre had received children who were under 16 and those aged between 16 and 17 had been placed in a centre run by Finding Your Feet. As noted above, this agency operated a service contracted in by the Social Services Department employing relatively unqualified or poorly qualified staff. Interviewees reported that the extension of the implementation of Section 20 to cover all children had a decisive effect in ushering in 'a whole new way of working' involving a higher degree of professional social worker involvement and more intensive procedures and monitoring.

The centre was very isolated geographically; was several miles from the nearest town and had a very poor local transport infrastructure. The boys who stayed there were generally positive about the treatment they received by staff and about the basic facilities offered to them. However, they did have clear expectations about access to education and later employment and the location of the centre presented serious obstacles to the prospect of attending schools or colleges. As with the unaccompanied minors and general asylum seekers referred to earlier, the boys had arrived with expectations of moving to London or surrounding areas and had little or no knowledge of other parts of the UK.

As it was not a compulsory scheme, staff needed to find volunteers from among the boys who would be willing to relocate to Manchester. They did this by discussing it initially with one boy and suggesting that he discussed it with his peers. This was followed by structured meetings in which various aspects of the proposal were presented. Social work staff at the centre, interviewed by the author, reported that one particularly strong 'selling point' was the potential educational opportunities that existed in the Manchester area and that staff assured the boys that they could go to colleges within days of arrival. Besides education, further pull factors reported by the social workers were the prospect of a shared house available for every two boys and the association of the city with Manchester United football team. A picture book was prepared by social services staff giving a view of the city including its considerable ethnic diversity, religious and cultural centres. Staff members were surprised that the image of people from a wide variety of ethnic backgrounds did not elicit uniformly positive responses from the boys. This aspect is returned to below.

Put briefly, the basic structure of the scheme was that after the boys arrived in Dover and followed the procedures described above, they were moved to the residential centre where they were offered a possible transfer to the Manchester area. The boys were placed under Section 20 of the Children Act and an assessment of their situation and social care needs was undertaken prior to their move. There was also some training provided in practical living skills aimed at equipping the boys to live semi-independent lives. Workers from the areas the unaccompanied minors were being transferred to visited them in the residential centre to familiarise themselves with the boys' living conditions prior to dispersal and to assess their capacity to undertake the move. Prior to the transfer, reception arrangements had been prepared in the Manchester area through extensive networking initiated by social services involving health services, education, recreational facilities and legal support. Of the 30 boys who were part of the pilot scheme, ten were placed in Manchester and a further ten were placed in each of two nearby towns. A child social worker and a full-time social care worker were assigned to each group of boys and they provided consistent ongoing support. In each of the areas the boys lived in pairs in five properties that were generally of good quality and a range of basic amenities including television, washing machines and second-hand computers were provided.

In investigating the situation of the boys in late 2005, it was apparent that much of the work that had been undertaken was genuinely motivated by concern for their welfare. The co-ordinated care associated with the status of being 'looked after' under Section 20 appeared to a certain degree to have been achieved. Basic needs for food, shelter and clothing had been provided to a reasonably high standard and the boys had access to weekly allowances in the region of £40. Legal services were engaged to ensure that a reasonable level of support and advice were offered for asylum claims. Groups were established, facilitated by social workers and supported by interpreters to explore with the boys what service providers felt were central issues in living in the UK. These included social inter-action, including interaction with members of the opposite sex and issues of sexual health. These sessions were unconsciously normative in their orientation and included messages about the 'correct' way to interact with people and to show respect to women. There was among the service providers a concern with sexual issues that appeared consistent with their general practice towards young people of a similar age. Interestingly, the boys responded to much of this with a mixture of bewilderment and embarrassment, for example, when they received 'welcome packs' that included a packet of condoms. Social workers reported that many of the boys seemed upset by this and threw the condoms away.

Contrasting perspectives on issues of sexuality between service provider and refugee clients have been noted by Ong in her study of social care services in the US targeted at Cambodian clients. Commenting on social worker practices relat-ing to Cambodian children, Ong has noted the prevalence of normalising discourses that seek to realign parents and children's practices with American val-ues. Within this context the highly controlled interactions between girls and boys promoted in traditional Cambodian families was viewed as a 'problem to be man-aged' by social work staff (Ong, 2003, p180). Similarly problematic encounters were frequently recorded between Western 'liberal' sexual values and the often more traditional values of refugee and migrant communities. A representative of a Somalian refugee organisation in Finland described the problems that arose when teenagers were automatically sent information packs on sexual health that included condoms, much to the consternation of many refugee parents and the teenagers themselves (personal communication).

Despite good intentions and careful forward planning, there were some areas of concern both to the boys themselves and to the service providers. These included a range of practical difficulties in terms of interpreting services. For example, when the boys went for health assessments they could often not com-municate with the GP and the only interpreting facility was through a telephone. There then ensued a complicated and awkward interaction on personal matters through this three-way dialogue. Often services were organised around nationali-ties or broad language groups that did not address significant regional and national variations and boys commented that although services engaged someone who was presented as speaking their language, they could not actually understand them. There were, for example, problems at various stages following arrival aris-ing from providing Dari interpreters for Pashto speakers (the two official languages of Afghanistan) and vice versa.

More broadly, there was a significant gap between, on the one hand, the boys' aspirations and expectations and the views of the service providers as to what would be appropriate for them. For service providers, there was a combi-nation of introducing normative arrangements and practices that reflected a desire to provide services generally viewed as appropriate for children of their age. These included giving information, group discussions and materials relat-ing to sexual health, referred to above. This general view of children's 'needs' also underpinned the provision of health assessments, access to recreational and sports facilities, the provision of computers and attempts to enrol them on college courses as quickly as possible. Alongside the view of unaccompanied minors as children requiring child-specific care and attention there was the view of them as constituting a very specific and distinctive group for whom a range of special measures were required. These special measures can be seen to consist of two groups of practices. Firstly, there were those that related to the boys as asylum seekers occupying a specific legal and political position and secondly there were what I refer to as culturally oriented measures or the 'cultural dimension' of care.

In what may be described as the political-legal dimension, the practices addressed towards the minors were directed specifically towards their position as unaccompanied asylum-seeking children. As noted above, efforts to provide social care were made alongside what can be called the 'immigration trajectory' that may be defined as the rules and practices governing their specific status as asylum seekers. This aspect placed particular constraints on the provision of social care, not least because of the possibility that the boys would be returned to their countries of origin when they reached 18. This dimension also manifested in the need to develop practical arrangements for the unaccompanied minors to have access to solicitors and advocacy services. Protocols were introduced aimed at ensuring that there was what was referred to as a 'transparent case transfer system' wherein a solicitor from the area of the port of entry would have their legal cases transferred to a solicitor in the Manchester area.

The 'cultural dimension' relates to those aspects of care aimed at addressing what were construed as the boys' specific cultural needs. It is also considered here as a two-way process in which the unaccompanied minors formulated their own needs in the British context. In practical terms, the cultural dimension here was manifest from the earliest stages of the minors' reception, informing areas such as the selection of interpreters, the food offered and facilities for religious observance. Within the safe case transfer process, the cultural dimension was also apparent in some of the strategies used to 'sell' Manchester to the boys, specifically in highlighting the ethnic, cultural and religious diversity in the city. In moving the boys, consideration was given to the presence and proximity of similar ethnic groups, religious and cultural centres. The identity and location of these centres was given to the boys in their welcome packs.

It is interesting that, while the importance of culturally appropriate care was stressed by the social workers and support staff, they simultaneously acknowledged that they felt they had little understanding of the cultural backgrounds of the boys and would welcome training in this area. Despite this, a number of assumptions were made about what would be culturally appropriate and helpful. Besides the provision of appropriate food, for example halal meat, it was assumed that the boys would feel more comfortable living in an ethnically diverse environment and close to a mosque and 'appropriate' cultural centre. These assumptions did not appear to be driven by views that had been expressed by the boys themselves but by a set of 'common-sense assumptions' deriving from the fact that they had come from Islamic countries. In fact, while some aspects of living in an ethnically diverse environment were welcomed, for example the availability of familiar food, some of the boys expressed disquiet at seeing black people and being treated by black service providers. They were particularly surprised when they found GPs and social workers from black and minority ethnic backgrounds, with one boy commenting that 'this is not what we expected in England'.

Service providers were very surprised after the first few months of the project to note that very few of the boys had gone to the mosque and fewer still had shown any interest in attending an Afghan community group. There was an expectation that they would behave in ways that were seen as 'culturally appropriate' and religious organisations in particular would be sought to find solace in a strange land and to connect with fellow believers. The boys, by contrast, were a little mystified by the assumption that they would be particularly religious and be enthusiastic to attend Afghan or other community groups. What service providers seemed unable to grasp fully was that they had paid a very high price physically, emotionally and financially to escape their countries and were driven by a strong vision of their life in England. Many had CDs and pictures of British and American pop stars with them when they arrived and, as one service provider observed, had some ideas of England that derived from Harry Potter films. They appeared to aspire to live with a 'normal' English family, go to school and college to be educated and then find a job. This remark by one boy was typical of the sentiments expressed in the group: 'I saw a lot of difficulties in my country, I want to become something. I don't want to be lazy and I want to be useful. I want to live life. I want to try hard in my new life'.

Their aspirations were generally unremarkable and entirely understandable. As with the children on the Spanish border, in Zeebrugge and across the industrialised world, they were fleeing unsafe environments in which they had little or no opportunities. As noted, there was 'no future' for these children in their countries of origin. The issue of achieving some form of cultural continuity with the traditions of their countries of origin was not a priority for the boys. Having said this, this statement requires more nuanced interpretation. When asked by service providers, the priority for the boys was clearly education and employment as well as a reasonable level of support while being educated. The relatively muted response to the availability of community groups and mosques was not because of a lack of interest in maintaining links with their own culture and languages, but rather because this was achieved primarily through strong personal relations with other boys from similar backgrounds, rather than through engaging with formal organisations.

As such, the boys' responses implicitly challenged essentialist views of their cultural needs. Service provider's responses were influenced by implicit and pervasive views of what constituted the boys' 'own community'. These views assumed a broad altruistic solidarity engendered simply through belonging to a similar religious or national group. Put very simply, the assumption was made that, as Muslims, the boys would feel most comfortable with other Muslims. As, say, Afghans, they would feel most comfortable with other Afghans. The assumptions were not based on discussions with the boys, or indeed with other service providers. It was simply 'obvious'. Underpinning this was a sense that they had, to some degree, lost their own cultures and identities and that part of the mission of social care agencies was to try and restore the boys' shattered worlds. Such a view is unsurprising as it is routinely presented in a range of publications and reports on the mental health and social care of refugees (CVS consultants, 1999).

The social anthropologist, Lisa Malkki, has argued that similar views are pervasive in the field of refugee studies and are influenced by an orientation within anthropological research towards the study of 'indigenous peoples', 'local contexts' and 'closed systems' as opposed to studying the movement and traffic of people. In refugee studies one finds again and again, 'the assumption that to become uprooted and removed from a national community is automatically to lose one's identity, traditions and culture' (Malkki, 1995b, p508). As many anthropological studies have testified, traditions are often maintained and transformed in countries and areas of resettlement in ways that strengthen a sense of allegiance towards a country and/or ethnic identity (Eastmond, 1998; Appardurai, 1996). However, this is rarely achieved in any simple way by aligning to institutions or organisations broadly reflective of religion or nationality.

Moreover, the cultural dimension suggests a field of enquiry encompassing both the refugee children's sense of their own culture and the policies and practices of social care agencies in locating and placing the children within specific groupings and related institutional and community contexts. The contact with the children who were part of the Safe Case Transfer project suggests that they had complex cultural worlds that included traditional norms and attitudes deriving from their countries and regions of origin along with a strong adopted culture deriving from Western artefacts and Western-inspired visions. Interestingly, they appeared not to be disposed towards living in a self-enclosed community consisting of people of similar religious or cultural backgrounds, the type of segregated community routinely criticised as an unfortunate, even dangerous bi-product of multiculturalism. The encounter between the boys and service providers is thus less a 'clash of cultures' than a mismatch between distinctive perspectives.

In this way the formulations of service providers are often not so much multiculturalist as examples of a 'plural monoculturalism' defined by Amartya Sen as existing in situations that support 'having two styles or traditions coexisting side by side, without the twain meeting' (Sen, 2006, p157). So much of contemporary multiculturalism focused less on dynamic processes of cultural interrelationships and more on promoting cultural singularity and atomism. The Safe Case Transfer project presented two contrasting approaches; on the one hand, an emphasis on teaching the unaccompanied minors about what were seen as British norms and values, particularly as applied to relations with the opposite sex and, on the other, promoting integration with what was imputed to be the boys' 'own community'. One strand of activity was oriented towards integration and another towards monoculturalism. A significant challenge that remained facing service providers was how they could develop a deeper sense of the boys' own cultural worlds and their own priorities.

Conclusion

This chapter has drawn on material illustrating the very fluid and dynamic situation facing refugee children at a port of entry and in their subsequent regimes of care. It has been argued that the political-legal context in which refugee children are received into industrialised countries represents a 'state of exception' as defined by Agamben (Agamben, 2005). The conflation of the terms, 'political' and 'legal' is itself illustrative of the dynamic and relentless penetration of the political domain into the formulation of laws and policies, in response to a recurrent sense of crisis fuelled by extensive media coverage. The social care of refugee children is here shown to be prey to the intrusion of new policies revealing the tension between immigration and welfare trajectories. This tension is manifest in relations between national and local government and tangibly present in ongoing battles over the allocation and transfer of resources. Within the UK the extension of Section 20 to cover older refugee children represents a significant expansion in the domain of social care and specifically the role of the social worker as central to the planning and delivery of care. This expansion of the welfare regime has given rise to renewed demands for resources and increasing pressures on local government.

The domain of law is, as such, itself a site of conflict between legal rulings driven by constantly shifting immigration laws and those resulting from considerations of the welfare of the child. The positioning of some refugee children within a specific legal context resulted in opportunities for the provision of care from relatively inexpensive staff groups and organisations operating at 'arm's length' from mainstream services. As noted, legal rulings relating to child welfare disrupted these arrangements and gave rise to new cost-driven strategies in which statutory requirements were met through processes of dispersal.

5 Education
Policy and practice

This chapter focuses on the provision of education to refugee children. It begins with a brief overview of the broad policy context including the worldwide 'Education for All' declaration. Two brief 'case studies' are then presented, one drawing on research into the education of Palestinian children in a refugee camp in Jordan and another offering an overview of educational development in one major refugee-producing country. These provide a background to an examination of the contemporary theory, policy and practice towards refugee children in industrialised countries. Particular attention is paid here to work on social capital, in recognition of its contemporary influence on both research and policy in the educational and immigration spheres. The chapter also addresses some of the tensions that may exist between approaches and resources linked to settled minority ethnic groups and recently arriving refugee children through the evocation of the concept of the 'limited good'.

The examination of the education of refugee children includes consideration of macro, meso and micro aspects; from laws and policies at international and national levels, to the formation of educational services through the interrelationship between key agencies at local levels. These give rise to a consideration of identifiable models that are emerging at the micro level of practice and of fruitful approaches towards service development in this area.

'Education for All'

There is considerable literature on the education of refugee children, much of it focused on the role of education in emergency situations. In the 1990 worldwide Education for All declaration, 155 countries agreed on a policy and a wide-ranging strategy for addressing the global challenges arising from deficiencies in educational provision. These challenges included high levels of illiteracy and poor access to educational resources, particularly for girls. Researchers from UNESCO noted that the declaration was highly significant as it was the first time senior policy makers and representatives from the world of education and civil society had 'agreed on a world strategy to promote universal basic education for children, and to reduce massive illiteracy rates among young people and adults especially women' (UNESCO, 1999). There is explicit reference in the declaration to the education of refugee children in Article 3 which refers to the removal of educational disparities for underserved groups including, 'refugees: those displaced by war, and people under occupation'. Despite this commitment to refugee children, evidence from emergency situations suggests that refugees may be frustrated in securing educational support. As Verdirame and Harrell-Bond argue, 'while for humanitarian organisations, education is the last priority in an emergency, for refugees it is among the first' (2005, p254).

International bodies such as UNESCO have sought to counter the potential to pay little attention to refugee children and those affected by emergency situations by a range of measures including the preparation of a series of thematic studies. These have provided evidence of the challenges faced in particular countries affected by war and the significant displacement of populations. A series of investigations referred to below draw attention to the fact that education, and the institutions that provide it, are significant factors in both the destruction and the potential reconstruction of societies, cultures and communities.

In many countries in the developing world the educational infrastructures are at best fragile. Class and economic differences in access to education are ubiquitous internationally but may be particularly evident in some countries, with schools being available only for those in the upper tiers of society. Besides lack of investment in schools, there may be an absence of a wider infrastructure necessary to ensure that children have learning opportunities. For example, children in townships and favellas may be compelled to work to alleviate family poverty and, where schools are available. Gender inequalities and social and cultural taboos frequently militate against the opportunity for girls to attend schools. Within emergency situations this fragility is all too apparent as facilities are stretched to breaking point. Schools may be deliberately targeted by enemy combatants as a convenient way to spread fear and disrupt vestiges of social cohesion. Within situations of conflict, schools may also be targets for the recruitment of child soldiers. Singer has observed that

> both state armies and rebel groups typically target the places where children will both be collected in the greatest number and are most vulnerable to being swept in. The most frequent are secondary schools or orphanages, where children of suitable size are collected in one place, but out of contact with their parents, who would try to spirit them away.
>
> (Singer, 2006, p58)

Schools are not only places where the basic skills of literacy and numeracy are taught, but additionally highly emotive symbols of a community's hopes for the future. They are social hubs in which children meet and play and parents share experiences. They may also hold a key to the enhancement of the family's future through equipping children with skills that have the potential to open a degree of economic well-being hitherto unknown. Their fragility in emergency situations stems from the high levels of social and economic stability they require to operate on a day-to-day basis. Buildings need to be maintained, teachers paid and learning resources provided. There must be a practical infrastructure for children to get to school in safety and a secure environment provided while they learn. Emergency situations are characterised by widespread disruption to economic functioning, heightened levels of threat to physical security and declining levels of social trust. In these circumstances, the fragile links that make school and educational processes possible are likely to be destroyed. The impact of this destruction goes well beyond a scenario in which children and young people are unable to go to school for a time. The aspirations of whole communities are likely to be shattered and whole generations will lose the chance for improving their lives.

Given the degree of social, political and economic stability required for schools to function, it is hardly surprising that schooling is likely to be severely disrupted in war-torn environments. Here social fissures symptomatic of emerging conflict often become apparent. Lynne Jones, in her moving account of children growing up in wartime Bosnia, describes situations in which Muslim children became increasingly ostracised from their Serbian classmates. Firstly, the Serbian children stopped playing with them. Then they started to leave the school altogether.

> Nina was ten and doing very well in her third grade. She had noticed that her Serb classmates were leaving. Every day there was a different reason: 'I have to go to the village. We are going to the seaside for a picnic. Please can I leave the class?' She wasn't bothered although things were a bit strange. Around her apartment block people had started guarding at night, she didn't know why...Only now everyone had gone from the apartment block except two or three Muslim families who lived there...
>
> (Jones, 2004, p23)

Jones describes, as far as possible from children's own perspectives, incrementally deteriorating situations in which there was a steady fragmentation of cohesion and trust. The gradual implosion of the children's social worlds was often witnessed with little or no adult explanation, as though trying to present reasons for the events would add to the children's burden of woes. Within this situation, school was a site of interethnic relationship sponsored initially by an overarching national government. The breakdown of the systemic ordering of the school mirrored wider societal disintegration and the emergence of potent forms of ethnic identity and solidarity. The fragmentation characteristic of the Bosnian conflict may indeed be characteristic of changing patterns of violence in which there is an increasing role of paramilitaries and organised crime. According to Held *et al.*, 'such groups use forms of violence that are often dispersed, fragmented and directed against civilians. They commit atrocities and rape, and mount sieges. They often aim to pursue a form of identity politics or ethnic exclusion' (Held *et al.*, 1999, p72). The consequent social erosion and chaos often defies attempts at clear-cut explanation and moral certainty. The tragic events at Beslan in 2004 reflect these shifting contours of conflict. Here Chechen separatists held schoolchildren hostage in an action that resulted in some 350 deaths.

The roles of the Russian military and the Chechens in the actions leading to the deaths remains a matter of contention. In an examination of the conflict, Tony Wood refers to 'a logic of escalating violence in which schoolchildren were pawns in a brutal exchange' (Wood, 2004).

For those refugee children who are under the protection of international aid agencies, the experience of education may give rise to an ongoing sense of conflict between the aspirations engendered through the educational programmes and those of the community at large. This conflict is illustrated by Jason Hart in his work on Palestinian children living in refugee camps established by the United Nations. He argues that children are often caught between homogenising discourses of aid agencies, on the one hand, or that of community representatives and parents, on the other. He argues that 'for the most part, researchers in the field of refugee studies have tended to share with humanitarian agencies and political leaders a lack of interest in the views expressed by refugee children' (Hart, 2004, p174).

A particular focus of Hart's research is educational provision to refugee children offered by the United Nations Relief and Works Agency (UNRWA). This agency was originally established in 1948 as the United Nations Relief for Palestinian Refugees and reflected humanitarian considerations less than, 'the emergence of the Palestinian problem as a prominent issue on the United Nations political agenda' (Zolberg *et al.*, 1989, p24). Within the agency, education has a central role and absorbs approximately 50 per cent of its budget. Zolberg contends that the emphasis on education reflected a central ideological concern of the agency in that it was 'designed to resolve the Middle East conflict by turning Palestinians into attractive economic assets in the eyes of the receiving states, so as to overcome their resistance to resettlement' (ibid.).

Within the contemporary situation, the emphasis on supporting Palestinians towards a 'brighter future' is central in UNRWA's educational programmes. These programmes include 'ten grades of primary and secondary level schooling as well as kindergartens, colleges and vocational training centres' (ibid., p170). Hart notes that in the publicity surrounding the programmes the refugee children are commonly shown in school and in the majority of pictures as either 'individual cases of need' or 'an undifferentiated mass of humanity, often attired in uniform clothing'. Accounts of the children's lives are 'narrowly restricted to their function as passive beneficiaries of UNRWA's assistance' (2004, p171). As such refugee children are represented in ways that are depoliticised and ahistorical, as individual subjects detached from communal life. One interpretation offered by Hart and some of the refugees he interviewed is that UNRWA is 'merely a means for containing and ultimately redirecting the aspirations of young Palestinians away from the notion of return (in any form) and towards a future as skilled migrant workers, dispersed throughout the Middle East region and beyond' (2004, p172). The education system as presented by Hart is devolved from historical narratives of the Palestinian people's struggles and focused on the practical development of skills leading to 'better futures'. As such, these views are consistent with Zolberg's observations on the role of the educational programmes.

While the children were stripped of communal identities within the educational system, these were simultaneously reinforced outside the system where the wider community viewed the refugee camp as a symbol of steadfastness and the struggle for return to the homeland. Those who realised the economic potential of the education system and left the camps were often seen as guilty of betrayal. The children themselves were thus highly symbolic of communal aspirations for return to the homeland and their departure for more successful lives elsewhere conveys a sense of an erosion of commitment to a communal future. As John Berger notes on a visit to Ramallah, for many of the children the immediate economic challenges faced by families added to the disincentives towards formal education,

> Most of the boys whose faces are on the walls were born in refugee camps, as poor as shanty towns. They left school early to earn money for the family or help the father with his job, if he had one.
>
> (Berger, 2003)

Refugee children were thus caught between an educational system that did not engage with traditional communal aspirations and a community within which there seemed little, if any, opportunities for future well-being. Furthermore, the images provided by the older generation of rural lifestyles had little attraction for young people in an urban refugee camp exposed to, 'a wide array of regional and global cultural products via satellite television, radio and film' (Hart, 2004, p178). A more potent influence for many was the ideology of Islamist movements that characterised Palestine as a land belonging to all Muslims and placed the battle for its repossession in a 'transhistorical' context. This provided a potential third route for generating and meeting the aspirations of young people.

Hart's analysis offers important insights not only into the specific instances he documents in a refugee camp in Amman, but also into wider questions about the role of education in refugee children's lives. It provides an example in which an education system is superimposed and governed by an ideology of individualism. Within this context, refugee children are faced with a choice between achieving self-fulfilment and a dream of communal regeneration through a return to lands of origin. The latter here may become denationalised and absorbed into a wider aspiration associated with the wider Muslim 'Umma', or community of believers.

Among the numerous questions raised here are those concerning the role education may play in providing social continuity through the teaching of communal history. The context of education here echoes Gramsci's distinction between classical and vocational education in which the latter is characterised by narrow instrumentality (Gramsci, 1971, p26). This instrumentality here precludes a contextualisation within which education is interlinked with the history and traditions of a community. Furthermore, the skills that are developed through the educational programmes have the impact not of developing their communities but of driving refugee children away to seek better lives elsewhere.

In some countries and localities, emergencies generating flows of refugees occur in situations in which educational systems in a Western sense have never reached parts of the population and, where they have, represent a relatively recent development. Education may predominantly take the form of skills and customs handed down from generation to generation. For example, in Somalia, nomadic pastoralists taught children the traditions of their clan and the skills and techniques required to survive. A more formalised system was introduced through Islam in which education was centred on the learning of the holy Koran. Among nomadic peoples, this teaching often followed their itinerant lifestyle with classes delivered in shaded outdoor areas and teachers paid directly by parents. The British and Italian colonial administrations introduced schools in the conventional Western sense after 1930 with the overarching aim of training clerical staff for the colonial administration. Education was, as such, conducted primarily in the languages of the colonisers (with some provision in Arabic) and the curriculum defined by what the colonisers viewed as important to support their enterprise. According to Bennaars and colleagues who undertook a review of progress in Somalia towards Education for All, 'towards 1960, the colonial system had produced only a handful of educated people and left a minimal education infrastructure. In short, colonial education appeared to be largely insignificant, if not irrelevant, to the vast majority of Somalis' (Bennaars *et al.*, 1996, p10).

A significant expansion of education occurred in the post-colonial period from the early 1970s, linked to the development of Somali as a written national language. This included the development of a mass literacy campaign aimed at all sections of society and a marked expansion in the numbers of teachers and children in primary schools. Rutter notes that 'by 1980 Somalia had a literacy rate of 60 per cent – no mean achievement in a country where about 60 per cent of the country are nomadic' (Rutter, 2003, p265). As Bennaars and colleagues record, the expansion was short-lived and, with the increasing emphasis on militarisation from the late 1980s, 'the formal education system collapsed almost completely. School buildings were being destroyed, educational material and equipment were being looted and teachers and administrators were not being paid' (1996, p12). The authors of the Education for All case study argue that the severe decline started prior to the civil war, the latter constituting a 'final blow' to the fragile system. It is instructive that a clear interrelationship could be identified between a rapid expansion in military spending and a decline in resources for education.

The example of Somalia has a number of salient features in common with that of other refugee-producing countries. Colonial administrations superimposed educational systems reflecting the values, traditions and interests of the colonisers. The language of the coloniser became the lingua franca of government, law and commerce; aspirations for improved status were inextricably bound to its mastery. However, the new social hierarchies allowed only elites from the colonised nations the opportunity to engage in the colonial administration. As Hobsbawm observes, the dynamics of the enterprise of empire in the twentieth century, 'consist essentially in the attempts by the elites...to imitate the model pioneered in the West, which was essentially seen as that of societies generating progress...' (Hobsbawm, 1994, p200). For the great masses, the indigenous languages remained pervasive and practical instruments of day-to-day interaction, but were often stripped of prestige and utility for the socially aspirant.

The languages, customs and traditions of the colonised were meanwhile systematised and rationalised by the coloniser in a manner conducive to European sensibilities. Moreover, they were harnessed to the enterprise of colonialism as forms of knowledge that would support the governance and exploitation of the population. Said, for example, in his seminal book *Orientalism*, refers to the processes through which the life of colonised lands were made intelligible by European writers and scholars; 'the eccentricities of Oriental life, with its odd calendars, its exotic spatial configurations, its hopelessly strange languages, its seemingly perverse morality, were reduced considerably when they appeared as a series of detailed items presented in a normative European prose style' (Said, 1978, p167).

The post-colonial era witnessed an immeasurable resurgence of pride in the languages and traditions, many of which were reinvented to fuel the aspiration for autonomy. Those fighting the colonial regimes often sought symbols that imbued the population with a sense of national solidarity, transcending religious and ethnic differences. For example, the Buddhist symbol of the wheel of dharma, the Asoka Chakra, was introduced as the centrepiece of the Indian flag. Asoka, a third-century Buddhist emperor, was famous for his tolerance and engagement with people of various faiths. While, at the time of independence, Buddhism was the religion of relatively few Indians, the symbolism was important precisely because it was not drawn from the two largest religions, Hinduism and Islam, but was associated with an image of a past that was both transcending sectarian divisions and was cultured and humane. Ironically, the architects of independence were normally from social elites often most distant from their fellow countrymen and women and closest to the coloniser. Commenting on the twentieth century, Hobsbawm observes that 'the history of the makers of the Third World transformations of this century is the history of elite minorities' (Hobsbawm, 1994, p202). These elites were necessarily familiar with the languages of the colonisers while the vast majority of the indigenous population were typically illiterate; some 90 per cent in the case of India at the time of independence. Furthermore, the ideologies that inspired the independence movements were Western, and often the products of these minority elites' familiarity with the languages and literatures of the colonisers.

In the post-colonial context, despite the emergence of local languages, many of the formerly colonised countries have maintained the languages of colonisers as the official lingua franca of government. English, for example, is the official language of Nigeria, Sierra Leone and Mauritius, while French is the official language of Niger, Gabon and Chad. Across South and Central America, Spanish and, in Brazil, Portuguese are dominant. Even where the languages of the colonisers have been replaced as the official language, they still often carry prestige and may be used within elite circles. Of the languages of the former colonial powers, English has become increasingly dominant. Held and his colleagues refer to it as standing 'at the very centre of the global language system', and as

> the central language of international communication in business, politics, administration, science and academia as well as being the dominant language of global advertising and popular culture. The main language of computing is English, providing the written language for Windows and Internet protocols.
>
> (Held *et al.*, 1999, p346)

Its dominance has made the learning of English of central concern to millions of people around the world seeking to improve their economic and social circumstances. Globally, English language learning is a central part of school curricula and represents a gateway to engaging in a world beyond regional or national boundaries. For refugee children arriving in the industrialised countries, this represents a particular pull factor towards the English-speaking countries, and partly explains the tendency to move to the UK from other potential countries of asylum.

Social capital and the education of refugee children

In many contemporary industrialised countries, education is routinely referred to in terms of investment in the future well-being and prosperity of the nation. In its broadest sense, however, education is simply one aspect of socialisation: it involves the acquisition of knowledge and the learning of skills. Thus, besides its centrality in ensuring long-term economic success, education is also generally seen, following Durkheim, as crucially important in securing social coherence and integration. According to him, 'Society can survive only if there exists among its members a sufficient degree of homogeneity; education perpetuates and reinforces this homogeneity by fixing in the child from the beginning the essential similarities which collective life demands' (1961). This is achieved through the transmission of society's norms and values necessary for social solidarity, the obeying of social rules and the positioning of children within the division of labour essential for economic productivity.

More recent educational theorists, notably Bourdieu, have analysed the role education plays in social reproduction through the perpetuation and enhancement of differentials of class and social status. Specifically, Bourdieu sought to identify the various 'mediations and processes' operating behind the backs of those directly involved in schools, pupils, teachers and parents, to 'ensure the transmission of cultural capital across generations and to stamp pre-existing differences in inherited cultural capital with a meritocratic seal of academic consecration' (Bourdieu and Passeron, 1990, pix). The school is, in other words, the site of an often-unconscious form of social reproduction while ostensibly providing an environment in which every pupil could achieve success purely on the basis of their abilities.

Bourdieu's contribution included the elaboration of concepts of capital, which he showed to be closely interrelated in perpetuating and legitimating social hierarchies. Eschewing the purely economic use of capital, he argued that 'capital presents itself under three fundamental species (each with its own sub-types), namely economic capital, cultural capital, and social capital' (Bourdieu and Wacquant, 1992, p119). Within Bourdieu's formulation, the study of these forms of capital was an attempt to reveal the tacit and implicit ways through which social hierarchies were maintained. By contrast, recent research emanating primarily from the US places a different emphasis on the analysis of social capital and one which may conform more closely to the earliest formulations of the concept (Putnam and Goss, 2002). Following the work of Hanifan from 1916, social capital is viewed as a concept decoupled analytically from other forms of capital. The emphasis in most recent scholarship has been on examining its role as a potentially key variable in a range of social and economic outcomes in spheres such as health, crime, ethnic relations, social cohesion and economic performance. Robert Putnam, one of the most prominent researchers in the field, describes social capital in the following terms: 'We describe social networks and the associated norms of reciprocity as social capital, because like physical and human capital (tools and training), social networks create value, both individual and collective, and because we can "invest" in networking' (Putnam and Goss, 2002, p4).

Much scholarship from the late 1980s has focused on the specific interrelationships between social capital and educational achievement (Coleman, 1988). While the foci of contemporary studies – the role of parents and communities in enhancing or undermining school achievement – would be familiar to educational researchers operating decades ago, the concept of social capital offers a neat encapsulation of a range of disparate elements. Put bluntly, work on social capital has highlighted the central role of relationships beyond that of the teacher–pupil in determining educational outcomes. What happens in the environment around the school is as critically important as the content of education itself, perhaps even more so.

Thus, studies have revealed the positive relationship between parents' educational achievements and engagement with their children's education and the latter's educational outcomes (Halpern, 2005, p142). Both 'structure' in the form of the number of adults and siblings in a household, and 'process' in the form of the level of interactions within the network, were positively associated with educational outcomes. This finding was particularly salient with respect to parents from higher-income categories. Children with both parents around fared better than those in one-parent families, possibly as a result of less interaction, but more likely related to a correlation with lower household income. More robust findings, based on the US National Educational Longitudinal Study of over 20,000 children, have shown that family mobility has a negative impact on educational achievement. According to Halpern, 'this implicates the importance of the wider social network on the child and parent. It is the disruption of this social capital external to the family itself that explains much of the relationship between family structure and educational outcomes' (Halpern, 2005, p147). A significant aspect of this social capital is encapsulated in the triadic relationship between parents, schools and children. Coleman argued that the relative success of students in Catholic schools in the US was a result of the shared values that exist between these three groups. In summarising Coleman's findings, Halpern comments; 'Catholic schools were associated with high levels of parent-school connectivity, and this appeared to be a key driving variable' (Halpern, 2005, p152).

Beyond evidence directly relating to the educational spheres, but highly relevant to the present topic, are findings relating to the lesser degrees of social trust that exist in multi-ethnic environments. Putnam alludes to this with reference to an unpublished study of social capital in 40 American communities which 'found that the problem of inequality in access to social capital is greatly exacerbated in socially heterogeneous communities'. He noted further with reference to this study,

> it appears that ethnic heterogeneity and high rates of immigration are part of the story. If so, then the rapid increase in ethnic immigration in most OECD countries in recent decades may pose important challenges to both the quality and social distribution of social capital in all our countries.
>
> (Putnam, 2002, p415)

Halpern makes the direct observation that 'there is considerable evidence that social and residential heterogeneity is associated with lower levels of social capital, not only between groups but within them'. And further, 'The higher the level of ethnic mixing within an area, the lower the level of social trust, associational activity and informal sociability' (2005, p260). Studies of the interrelationship between groups within this area often employ a conceptual distinction between 'bonding' and 'bridging' social capital, with the former relating to social capital developed between members of an ethnic group, and 'bridging' capital relating to the links made across ethnic groups. Research suggests that, where ethnic groups have strong 'bonding' social capital, they are likely to build bridges with other groups.

The social capital literature has been highly influential in the development of public policies, particularly in the US and the UK where it has a marked impact on the refugee field. In the UK, the National Integration Strategy for refugees employs the concepts of bridging and bonding social capital as indicators of the achievement of integration (Ager and Strang, 2004). The appeal of social capital research, with its emphasis on the development of social engagement, networks and trust, is considerable. Within the sphere of education, it has the potential to highlight the importance of recognising the wide range of influences that may impinge on the realisation of a child's potential and draw attention to the importance of close engagement between the school, parents and the wider community. However, the work gives rise to a number of issues pertinent to both the spheres of migration and refugees, and requires critical scrutiny.

Most fundamentally, as indicated above it is important to acknowledge that there is a marked shift of emphasis between the work of Bourdieu and that of Putnam, Coleman and numerous other scholars who have joined the field in the 1990s and

2000s. Bourdieu's work may be described as essentially critical in orientation and aims to expose the social relations that perpetuated economic and social inequality. Putnam's work, and that which has been influenced by him, is evaluative in orientation and treats social capital as a social 'good', present to greater or lesser degrees in different communities and individuals. High levels of social capital are equated with positive social outcomes including educational success, good health, low crime and harmonious community living. Within what may be referred to as the 'Putnam school', the emphasis is not only on identifying the impact of social capital but on promoting strategies to enhance its presence. This effort has displayed the characteristics of a missionary zeal and has included various high-level discussions with senior politicians including President Bush and Prime Minister Blair (Hallberg and Lund, 2005).

On an international level certain countries are identified as having more or less social trust and this is in turn related to a range of further indicators of social well-being (Putnam, 2002). Unsurprisingly, the countries recorded with the lowest levels of social trust (measured by the percentage agreeing that 'most people can be trusted') are among those with the highest levels of social inequality, with Brazil the lowest followed by a range of Latin American and African countries. The three countries with the highest levels of social trust are the Scandinavian countries of Denmark, Sweden and Norway respectively (Putnam, 2002). One significant feature is the correlation drawn by Putnam and others between social homogeneity, trust and social capital. The Scandinavian countries are generally seen as exemplary in the development of social capital and in reaping its benefits across a spectrum of areas. Sweden has been eulogised for its high participation in voting, volunteering, participation in informal study groups, informal socialising and, in contrast to the US, growing levels of social trust (Halpern, 2005, p218). Putnam assesses Sweden as ranking 'at or near the top' with respect to these aspects from a global perspective (Putnam, 2002, p395).

As indicated above, the high correlation between homogeneity and social capital is matched by findings indicating that high levels of ethnic diversity correlate with low social capital. More precisely, according to Hallberg and Lund, 'what Putnam has been perceiving for some time is the negative correlation between ethnic diversity, on the one hand, and community cohesion and social trust, on the other (2005, p58). At the time of writing, the full findings underpinning this perception remain unpublished and have emerged primarily instead in the context of small-scale seminars. However, these have often included senior politicians and policy makers and, as such, have influenced public concern and debate. It is too early to assess the impact of Putnam's diversity hypothesis, but it is reasonable to suggest that it has strengthened the position of policy makers sceptical of multiculturalism. One concern is that many of Putnam's conclusions in this area derive from research conducted in localities in the US, and require considerable caution in terms of assessing general validity. Bourdieu himself pointed to an unfortunate tendency to generalise from findings derived from the socio-historical particularities of the US (Bourdieu and Wacquant, 1999). Emerging findings from the UK, for example, suggest that a negative correlation between social capital and ethnic diversity cannot be easily drawn and the picture is complex. Recent findings have pointed to closer demographic integration of ethnic groups, a comparatively high level of mixed marriages and relationships, improving social attitudes to diversity and marked improvements in school performance of some ethnic groups (Kyambi, 2005; Page, 2006; Owen, 2004; Simpson, 2006).

A further concern regarding the formulation and deployment of the concept is that it suggests a form of society comprised of a largely homogeneous community with high potential for integration, which may be undermined by the presence of minority ethnic groups. The latter groups are themselves construed as potentially homogeneous and requiring 'bonding' to secure their cohesiveness and their potential to integrate successfully with the host community. One element that is ignored is that host societies that are homogeneous are so by virtue of a social and economic marginalisation of those construed as 'other'. The Netherlands and Scandinavian countries cited by Putnam and Halpern are noted for the high levels of unemployment among minority ethnic groups, low school achievement and high levels of housing segregation (Pred, 2000; Vasta, 2006). Interestingly, a notable phenomenon of the mid-1990s onwards has been the significant movement of Somalis who had achieved EU citizenship from the Netherlands and Scandinavian countries to the UK in an effort to improve their life chances (Watters, 2007).

It is perhaps helpful here to reflect briefly on the relationship between what Stuart Hall has referred to as the dialectic between 'belongingness and otherness' (1992). Fukuyama, among others, has noted that 'group solidarity in human communities is often purchased at the price of hostility towards out-group members'. He posits that a useful way of examining the externalities to social capital is through the concept of a 'radius of trust', 'that is the circle of people among whom cooperative norms are operative. If a group's social capital produces positive externalities, the radius of trust can be larger than the group itself' (Fukuyama, 1999, p2). Conversely, externalities that are negatively construed produce a constricted radius of trust. It is indeed notable that the countries identified as having high levels of trust have high degrees of ethnic homogeneity and racialised minority ethnic groups that are largely on the periphery of society. Specifically, Denmark, Sweden and the Netherlands have been identified among the high trust countries. The correlation between high national levels of trust and ethnic group marginalisation is a potentially fruitful area for further research.

Moreover, the arguments developed in relation to social capital and diversity are often implicitly based on a representation of individuals as having an identity defined primarily by their cultural or ethnic group. As argued previously, they may, as such, be characterised as underpinned by notions Amartya Sen has described as 'plural monoculturalism', in which cultural or racialised groups are clearly demarcated and identified primarily on the basis of their presumed difference. Sen's characterisation is one in which ethnic and cultural groups are treated as though they were entrenched and deeply determining of individual values and behaviour, with society consisting of a mosaic of self-contained units within which Durkheimian notions of altruistic solidarity prevail (Watters, 1996b). Sen points out that if multiculturalism is defended in the name of cultural freedom, then it can hardly be seen as demanding unwavering and unqualified support for staying steadfastly within one's inherited cultural tradition...no matter how important multiculturalism is, it cannot lead automatically to giving priority to the dictates of culture above all else.

(Sen, 2006, p158)

More specifically, recent formulations of the concept of social capital have particular implications for refugee children. The notion that increasing diversity diminishes social capital suggests significant challenges to schools seeking to incorporate refugee children from diverse ethnic backgrounds. The implication from Putnam's emerging research is that the social glue that maintains the links between parents, teachers and students will be loosened through the introduction of children from other cultural backgrounds. The view that building bonding social capital provides linkages between members of the same group and may be a prerequisite for the establishment of bridging social capital, presents a further challenge to refugee children. Unlike settled minority ethnic groups, refugees often have had little time to settle in a country and, particularly for those arriving as asylum seekers, are typically from a wide range of ethnic and cultural backgrounds. Schools accommodating refugee children often have small numbers from a wide diversity of backgrounds. The literature on social capital implies that a school with, say, a small number of children from, say, former Yugoslavia, Somalia, Iraq and Afghanistan would be faced with serious problems not only in terms of the impact on the children from the host society, but also in terms of the interrelationships between the refugee children themselves.

The literature on education and social capital suggests further that refugee children will be severely disadvantaged in terms of the external supports necessary to do well at school. Those living with parents are unlikely to be well integrated into the community and have established social networks. Many parents will themselves not speak the language of the host society and may even rely on the children for help with it. This suggests that parents are likely to find it very difficult to be involved in the schools provided by the host societies. This difficulty may extend to being unable to help children with homework, to engage in parent–teacher consultations and to participate in school-governing bodies.

A further challenge lies in the potentially deleterious effects of high levels of physical mobility among refugee children. The frequency of physical moves has been negatively correlated with educational achievement (Halpern, 2005, p157). Refugee children frequently enter schools in unsystematic ways, often at midpoints in the school year. Their integration into schools may be further disrupted by wider uncertainties regarding legal aspects such as their asylum application and policies of dispersal. Interestingly, the social capital literature indicates that even students with high-residential mobility and low social networks will benefit from being in areas where there are generally good links between parents, schools and the wider community. However, this potential benefit may be undermined by the placing of refugee children in schools where there are large numbers of mobile and marginalised families and in areas where there has been what has sometimes been referred to as 'white flight', whereby members of the host community have withdrawn their children from schools with high numbers of children from minority ethnic groups (Vasta, 2006).

A further issue suggested by the social capital literature is the potential for children who are seen as a problem to effectively 'live up to expectations'. Halpern cites a study by Defty and Fitz-Gibbon involving 120 'underaspiring' children in the UK who were identified as a group with specific needs and accorded additional pastoral support. Despite the additional support given to them, this group performed significantly worse in national exams than a control group that was not identified as having additional needs. Halpern concludes that 'this result is in line with much earlier studies showing that identifying a child as less able can affect teacher expectations and lower performance, and hence that individual interventions to prevent delinquency can actually lead to worse outcomes' (Halpern, 2005, p151). Anderson, in a study of refugee children in Germany, stresses that children feel that the quality of interaction with teachers is very important,

> the children revealed very sensitive antennae as regards the teacher's behaviour towards them, especially at the beginning. It was important that teachers showed themselves to be welcoming, but without drawing too much attention to the children's difference from their fellow pupils.
>
> (2001, p191)

This issue of identification of difference and/or special needs is important for refugee children who are routinely placed in visible and explicit contexts where they are given additional support.

The influential social capital literature would suggest that refugee children are thus likely to face severe difficulties in adapting to schools in the industrialised world. The much-vaunted close interactions between students, teachers and the schools are often simply not present for refugee children and there are additional problems relating to an absence of social networks, high mobility, poverty, placement in underperforming schools and the impact of being identified as 'problem' children. Further problem areas that have been identified include racism and bullying, interethnic violence and conflict (Rutter, 2006, p135). Indeed, an assessment of the various ways in which refugee children may fall short of a desired standard of care and support, both inside and outside of the school, is likely to provoke the conclusion that they are faced with intractable problems.

Rutter's extensive work on the education of refugee children would appear to support this perspective. Unlike much of the work done on school achievement, it draws clearly on a sample of refugee children as opposed to more generalised groupings on 'immigrant children'. In 2002, Rutter undertook an analysis of the examination records of 432 refugee children in the UK from Congolese, Somali and Turkish (Kurdish) backgrounds. The children were from a total of five different schools and the study included children who had been in the UK for less than five years. On the basis of her data, Rutter concluded, 'these children appeared to be underachieving in relation to other minority groups, including children of African-Caribbean and Bangladeshi origin, as well as white UK and Irish children' (Rutter, 2006, p137). There were, however, interesting variations in the findings. The results for the refugee children were by no means uniform with some groups, for example, the Congolese, doing significantly better than Somalis or Kurdish children in national tests. Rutter also alludes to the fact that, while in 2002, no Somali children in any of the schools had achieved five GCSEs graded A to C, in one of the schools 36 per cent of Somali children had achieved this score by 2004. She also notes that among relatively recently arrived children from southern Sudan the majority 'were making progress comparable to, or better than the targets expected of average British children' (2006, p203).

Thus, underpinning what appears as a remorselessly negative situation, there is evidence of some groups of refugee children managing, to some degree, to transcend adversarial circumstances. In her description of the school where Somalis achieved a significant improvement in their results, Rutter noted that it was a school chosen by refugee parents despite having a generally poor reputation. The parents believed their children would receive the necessary support to enable their children to progress, and the evidence suggests that many made an astute judgement. Rutter remarks that, as such, there is evidence of refugee parents exercising choice in ways that challenge prevailing 'assumptions that only middle class parents possess agency and the means to exercise choice in education' (ibid., 2006, p134). It may be noted that refugees themselves are often from middle-class backgrounds and were well educated within their countries of origin. Indeed, as Van Hear has argued, refugee diasporas are themselves closely related to considerations of class and income, with social and economic capital determining the degree to which many refugees can flee their countries and regions of origin (Van Hear, 2006). Those reaching European and other industrialised countries are often those with relatively reasonable reserves of income and social networks. This is not, of course, to suggest that refugees in the industrialised countries are 'well off', as the resources they had are often spent in attempting to escape across international borders. However, an emphasis on agency here is important as the efforts of refugee children and their families are a critical aspect in achieving a measure of success. A number of commentators have noted that refugees generally place a strong emphasis on education and this may be reflective of the fact that they do not have other mechanisms for social advancement through, for example, family networks. Halpern makes the broad point that, 'while the affluent and well connected can build a successful career on their connections, those from disadvantaged, less well connected families instead must concentrate on attaining academically' (Halpern, 2005, p149).

In sum, the social capital literature does present important research questions and areas for investigation. It supports the extensive evidence that links social circumstances of children and families with their performance at school. Beyond this, it offers insights into the effects of parent–child and parent–school relationships in influencing educational achievements. While helpful in suggesting questions that should be considered in relation to the education of refugee children, an emphasis on social capital alone is unlikely to be satisfactory in explaining the variations in school performance and experiences of refugee children. It is notable that in countries that score highly on social capital the performance of children from black and minority ethnic groups can be very poor. The social factors that promote cohesion among the host community appear related negatively to a tendency towards the 'othering' of those who are from the outside.

Furthermore, evidence suggests that achievement is a 'two-way street' requiring a combination of refugee agency and resilience and the simultaneous creation of opportunities by the schools and education authorities. Bearing this in mind, it is useful analytically to distinguish between three levels of activity that act on the capacity of refugee children and their families to fulfil their potential in the sphere of education. These may be identified as follows:

1   At a macro or institutional level, the policies developed by international bodies, national and local governments that impinge on refugee children's education. These include, for example, the impact of legislation relating to education generally and specific policies relating to families and children from minority ethnic groups. This level also includes legislation and policies relating to asylum and immigration.

2   At a meso level of local implementation, the policies and practices developed by schools and education authorities in relation to refugee children. These policies and practices may be embedded in wider policies towards ethnic minority or immigrant children.

3   At a micro level, the interaction between 'service providers' – whether teachers, school governors, counsellors, health or social care staff – and refugee children. The roles of these staff should not be seen as merely 'instrumental', but as actively involved in the interpretation and implementation of policy within the institutional constraints imposed upon them. They are, as such, to borrow again Lipsky's expression 'street level bureaucrats' who deliver services in distinctive ways (1980).

These levels may all be seen as spheres of engagement for refugee children or for those agencies that seek to support and represent them. Thus, for example, refugee children and their families may be largely confined to the micro level in exercising agency, through engagement with, say, teachers. Organisations that lobby on their behalf may exercise influence on the meso and macro levels. They in turn may (and indeed should) draw on direct interaction with refugee children and families in pressing for official bodies to meet their needs and assure their rights. Furthermore, the levels should not be seen as simply operating in a 'top down' manner in any straightforward way. Events at meso or micro levels could have a bearing on the development of laws and policies through, for example, attempting to spread 'good practice' emanating from initiatives developed at a local level. This is likely to emerge in situations where a degree of local autonomy is countenanced or even encouraged.

In sum, while the division of activity in this sphere into macro, meso and micro levels may appear excessively formulaic, I would argue that it is useful in three ways. One is that it demonstrates the embeddedness of practices within legal, policy and funding contexts. Second, it draws attention to the interrelationships between policy and practice and third, it can help demonstrate the movement between the levels suggesting both 'top-down' and 'bottom-up' processes. As such, the approach here avoids the dualism identified by Giddens where 'micro-situations' are those to which a notion of agency is appropriate, whereas 'macro-situations' are those over which individuals have no control. Rather, the approach here accords with Giddens' view that 'what is important is to consider the ties, as well as the disjunctions, between situations of co-presence and "mediated connections" between individuals and collectivities of various types' (Giddens, 1993, p7). The meso level, as proposed here, represents a means to identify mediated connections between institutional policies and processes and refugee children.

Macro level: international treaties and directives

The education of refugee children is appropriately considered in the context of the various physical, social and legal positions in which refugee children are placed. It is difficult to speak in any meaningful way about the topic without taking broader factors into account. For example, access to, and experience of, education is likely to be significantly affected by asylum status and the broad legal and policy framework in which children are received. If they arrive in the industrialised countries as part of an organised and agreed programme of resettlement, children are likely to be treated with a degree of forward planning tailored towards their needs. They will probably be incorporated within mainstream schools, perhaps with specialised classes aimed at improving their language skills, and given induction programmes aimed at wider integration into the host society. For those arriving in industrialised countries as asylum seekers, whether in family groups or alone, access to education is likely to be considerably more difficult to achieve. In many receiving countries, children are placed in reception centres or detention and, consequently, the education they receive is outside of mainstream provision.

The UN Convention on the Rights of the Child Article 28 confirms that every child has a right to education and this right should be progressively achieved through compulsory and free primary schooling. The United Nations General Assembly Special Session on Children in 2002 produced a document entitled, 'A World Fit for Children'. Paragraph 7(5) of the declaration states, 'All boys and girls must have access to and complete primary education that is free, compulsory and of a good quality as a cornerstone of an inclusive basic education' (cited in Antoniou and Reynolds, 2005, p153). The 1951 convention relating to the status of refugees affirms in Article 22 the responsibility of the government of the country of asylum to provide education for refugees (UNHCR, 1994). The UNHCR Executive Committee in 1992 asked that, 'the basic primary education needs of refugee children be better addressed and that, even in the early stages of emergencies, educational requirements be identified so that prompt attention may be given to such needs' (UNHCR, 1992). In its formal guidelines, UNHCR stresses the importance of school in promoting the overall well-being of children: 'Attending school provides continuity for children, and thereby, contributes enormously to their well-being. For these reasons, education is a priority in terms of protection and assistance activities' (UNHCR, 1994).

Across the industrialised countries there appears to be a general convergence of perspectives regarding refugee children's rights to education as reflected in national standards and guidelines on good practice. For example, the 'best practice' guidelines for separated children in Canada prepared by the International Bureau for Children's Rights contains the following statement on access to education: 'Separated children, irrespective of their immigration status, should have access to the same statutory education as national children. Separated children should have full access to all services within schools, including the services of school social workers and counsellors' (International Bureau for Children's Rights, p30).

It is important here, as in other areas of policy relating to refugee children, to distinguish between law, policy, good practice guidelines and actual practice 'on the ground'. While many good practice guidelines and standards set by leading NGOs clearly stress the importance of refugee children having the same rights to education and associated provisions as native children, official policy directives and laws may subtly allow for the development of distinctive provisions. For example, the European Union Council Directive of 2003, laying down minimum standards for the reception of asylum seekers, states in Article 10 on the 'schooling and education of minors' that:

> Member states shall grant to minor children of asylum seekers and to asylum seekers who are minors access to the education system under similar conditions as nationals of the host Member State for so long as an expulsion measure against them or their parents is not actually enforced. Such education may be provided in accommodation centres.
>
> (European Commission, 2003)

It is notable that the wording refers here not to the same provision but to access 'under *similar* conditions to nationals' (my italics) and allows for the provision of education within accommodation centres. The article goes on to stipulate that where access to the education system is not possible owing to the 'specific situation of the minor, the Member State may offer other educational arrangements'. There are no examples or guidance given here as to what these situations may be or of the range or standards of the alternative arrangements. One seemingly unambiguous aspect of the directive is the responsibility of member states to provide access to the education system within three months of the application for asylum. However, even here there is allowance for the period to be extended to one year where 'specific education is provided in order to facilitate access to the education system'. A critical reading of the article may thus suggest that refugee children receive different provision to nationals, that they can be educated outside of mainstream schools, that it is at the discretion of the member state as to whether the 'situations' of the minors call for alternative provision, and member states can withhold access for up to a year where it is deemed appropriate by them to offer some unspecified alternative provision.

Under Article 26 of the directive, the member states of the European Union were required to bring into force 'laws, regulations and administrative provisions' necessary to comply with it. The broadly construed and capacious formulations of the article make it difficult to see how they might seriously act to improve practice in the area of education. The directive represents a key component in the creation of a Common European Asylum System, an objective set out by the European Council in Tampere, Finland in 1999, an aspect of which is the harmonisation of conditions for the reception of asylum seekers.

Within the parameters of the directive however, there appear to be considerable disparities in terms of educational provision between member states. For example, in Denmark – which opted out of the Directives, but has sought to develop policies consistent with it – asylum-seeking children do not have the right to enter the state educational system and are, instead, placed in classes provided by the Red Cross which runs 12 special schools for this purpose. Children who have been in Denmark for over 12 months may be allowed to join the state system but these places are specially funded by the Red Cross (UNHCR, 2005). As such, the Danish system accords with the terms of the directive insomuch as asylum-seeking children can be seen as those requiring up to 12 months of special provision before entry into mainstream schools. Here however, their marginality is perpetuated by the existence of special funding arrangements for their education.

Further disparities exist in terms of the institutional location of educational provision in that, in many European countries, primary education is provided within the context of 'accommodation centres' and refugee children do not go to mainstream schools. Indeed there are wide disparities that can be charted across an axis of integration and separation. In Belgium, for example, children of primary school age are integrated into mainstream schools with some special provision for Dutch language education (within the Flemish areas). The regional government provides funding on a per capita basis for the latter. By contrast, at a secondary level, non-Dutch speaking minors are offered intensive language courses for a period of 12 months in special reception classes. The children go to school but are segregated within the school system for one year. Only schools with at least 25 migrant newcomers receive special government finance to enable them to run these special classes, so within particular areas schools agree where the migrant children will be allocated and the special classes run. The children's school week consists of 22 hours of special language teaching, two hours on religion and morals and a further four hours that can be arranged at individual schools' discretion (Mels and Derluyn, 2006).

There is as such a high level of management control over the education received by refugee children. The centralisation of resources ensure that children or their families exercise little choice over where they go to school and the curriculum is largely centrally prescribed and determined. The situation is further differentiated in the Netherlands where a large majority of all children located within the asylum determination procedure receive their education within or close to special accommodation centres. Much of this provision centres on the Dutch language teaching and cultural instruction. In terms of primary education, each accommodation and asylum-seeker centre has its own school that provides intense Dutch language training for one year before children are transferred to regular primary schools. According to de Ruuk, in some cities there are no special schools for asylum-seeking children and they are immediately transferred into mainstream schools. Reporting on the situation in 2001, no less than 10,000 refugee children attended primary schools in the asylum-seeking centres where they were placed or in the neighbourhood of the centre. Eighty per cent of the children stay at the school for between one and two years while the others can stay for periods of over two years (de Ruuk, 2002).

Children aged between 12 and 18 go to mainstream Dutch secondary schools, but are generally placed in special classes known as ISC, International Switch Classes. While children who have spent over 12 months in a Dutch primary school are allowed to go to classes with their Dutch peers when they reach secondary school, in practice many appear to be allocated to ISC classes until the end of their school education. The situation in the Netherlands thus similarly excludes children by keeping them outside of the mainstream system. They exist in largely liminal situations in which the insecurity of their asylum situation is compounded by an existence within self-contained institutional contexts. The emphasis of the school curriculum is on ensuring a one-way process of adaptation or assimilation through language and cultural training. The situation in Sweden displays basic similarities in that asylum-seeker children will go to separate introduction classes in their first year of school.

The above examples are illustrative of the fact that, while some countries ensure an entitlement to education and thus ostensibly comply with the EC Directive, there is in fact a clear differentiation in the provision for children at least while they are within the asylum system. This differentiation relates to a broader consideration of the position of refugee children with respect to the welfare and the immigration trajectory. The exclusion of children from mainstream schools is not only an exclusion from educational instruction but also from the wider benefits that potentially accrue in terms of socialisation and integration. In the Belgian system, schools are developed that specialise in migrants – a process that is underpinned by the funding mechanisms created by the government. While creating some schools that offer specific services for migrants, the system simultaneously creates schools that exclude them. Schools with high numbers of migrants are shunned by some parents from the autochthonous population who, following the arrival of migrant children, seek to move their children elsewhere. As observed previously, Vasta has noted this phenomenon in the Netherlands; 'there appears to be a process of "white flight" from schools with high numbers of immigrant children' (Vasta, 2006, p11). Dench and colleagues have likewise noted some parallel processes in the UK (Dench *et al.*, 2006). A further interesting effect that will be discussed below is that refugee children's parents sometimes view the high concentration of migrant children as being detrimental to the integration of their children (Mels and Derluyn, 2006).

In the UK, the policy has been to integrate asylum-seeking children into mainstream schools as quickly as possible. In 2003 there was an estimated 98,929 asylum-seeker and refugee children in schools across the UK (Arnot and Pinson, 2005, p4). The legal context for their education is provided by Section 14 of the Education Act 1996, which requires local authorities to provide education for all children aged between 5 and 16, including children of asylum seekers and refugees. Asylum-seeking children are normally placed within local schools and those in the care of social services departments are required to receive a full-time education placement in a local school within 20 school days. The Education Act 2005 took this latter requirement a step further and made it a statutory responsibility to prioritise school admissions of 'looked after' children, a category that included many unaccompanied asylum-seeking children. Local Education Authorities were required (but did not always accomplish) to provide additional educational support in this category including a personal education plan and a responsibility on schools to designate a named person to co-ordinate the child's educational provision (Free, 2005, p35).

As these examples suggest, it is important to be mindful of the potential distinction that may exist between entitlement and access. Entitlement refers to the right, enshrined in law and policy, to receive a service, while access here refers to the practical process through which refugee children actually enter a service. As such, the concepts have referents at a macro level at which law and policy are formulated and at a micro level at which they are implemented. Access by contrast can only be properly analysed with reference to local situations in which refugee children enter schools. As noted above, with respect to the situation in the UK, one further salient macro-level factor is the policy of dispersal whereby asylum seekers have been moved away from the densely populated and expensive south east of England to the Midlands and the North where housing is cheaper and more readily available. This policy has had a significant impact on educational provision in that areas with hitherto little experience of receiving asylum seekers or children with similar ethnic backgrounds faced the challenge of incorporating the children into local schools. The UK National Children's Bureau (NCB) reported that the majority of children present themselves in the middle of school terms and, in practice, 'it can take weeks or months to find a school place and then often only in the lowest performing schools' (Appa, 2005, p7). Thus, while the *entitlement* to receive school education may be met, *access* to education is hindered by the impact of immigration policies on refugee children.

Ethnic minority and refugee children: the image of the limited good

One salient issue with respect to the education of refugee children and indeed to other aspects of social welfare, is the extent to which policies and practices derive from broader approaches established in relation to settled immigrant communities. Some academics and service providers have argued that the challenges and struggles faced by refugees closely parallel those faced by settled black and minority ethnic communities and a common approach should be adopted where possible. For example, in commenting on mental health service provision, Fernando argues that 'refugees should not be seen as a separate group but as basically a part of the groups we call ethnic minorities' (Fernando, 2005, p184). This view is implicitly echoed in the construction of various guides for practitioners that incorporate both strategies for meeting the needs of ethnic minority children and those of refugee children (e.g. Dwivedi, 2003).

The issues here are complex and need to take into account the social, legal and political context. As noted above, in many countries refugee children are placed in very specific institutional contexts in terms of the provision of services such as health care, accommodation and education. These often severely restrict their or their families' autonomy and place them in a highly marginal position in relation to mainstream services. A further complexity is that the presence of a large majority of settled minority ethnic groups may reflect the vagaries of colonial histories, whereas refugees are likely to be from a very highly diverse range of countries, spanning continents and with a wide range of religious and ethnic backgrounds.

In practice, it is probably unhelpful to construct the discussion in a dichotomised manner suggesting that there is some ultimate choice to be made between incorporating or not incorporating refugees within wider initiatives for minority ethnic groups. Put simply, it depends on the service and on the group in question. A mental health strategy, for example, developed for a settled community of Sikh Punjabis is unlikely to reflect the needs of newly arrived refugees from Eastern Europe living in reception centres. On the other hand, one could envisage initiatives developed for, say, settled Congolese communities in Belgium providing a potentially useful basis for the development of services for Congolese refugees. Furthermore, in addressing issues of racism and discrimination, initiatives developed towards settled minority communities may provide useful guidance for developments in services for some refugee groups. However, it should not be assumed that refugees would necessarily feel part of, nor wish to participate in, generalised strategies towards black and minority ethnic groups. At the level of policy and practice, the tensions that may exist between service provision for minority ethnic groups and refugees can be illustrated with reference to developments in education in the UK.

The interaction between educational and immigration laws and policies and their impact on the schooling of refugee children is illustrated by Jill Rutter, education advisor to the Refugee Council between 1988 and 2001. In an analysis of the UK context since the mid-1980s she describes refugee children's education as affected both by immigration processes and law and policy relating to black and minority ethnic groups. Prior to the beginnings of recognition of the specific needs of refugee children in the early 1990s, funding was only available for refugee children through diverting funds made available through Section 11 of the Local Government Act 1966. This funding was identified for 'immigrants from the Commonwealth whose language and customs differ from those of the community' (Local Government Act, 1966). In the late 1980s, around 82 per cent was used in education, mostly to provide English Additional Language teaching in schools (Rutter, 2006, p108). It was not, as such, designed to meet the needs of refugee children. Rutter records that in 1988, 'local authorities used Section 11 to employ teams of teachers who were seconded to particular schools, or formed peripatetic teams'. These serviced refugee children from Iran and Eritrea with local authorities turning a 'blind eye' to the requirement that the target population should be from the Commonwealth (ibid.).

Rutter records the attempts made by refugee advocacy groups through the late 1980s and early 1990s to extend the scope of Section 11 funding to include provision for all minority ethnic groups, a goal that was eventually achieved in 1993. Influential groups supporting the rights of black and minority ethnic groups who viewed the funding as vital for anti-discriminatory and 'race' equality work opposed the extension of funding to refugees. According to Rutter, 'when a group of white European refugees arrived, their eligibility for Section 11 funding was questioned because of their lack of blackness'. These tensions 'highlighted the split between the advocacy coalitions concerned with refugee children and those concerned with British minority ethnic communities' (Rutter, 2006, p114). There was some resolution to this conflict when these disparate coalitions united against government-initiated moves to replace Section 11 in the mid-1990s.

In 1998, following a government review, the Ethnic Minority Achievement Grant (EMAG) replaced Section 11 monies. In line with a more general devolution of funding from local authorities to schools, local authorities could retain only 15 per cent of the funds with the remainder going directly to school budgets. As Rutter observes, the sums made available under the EMAG were about two-thirds of £130 million or so provided under Section 11. However, the introduction of the grant did have the merit of creating a consolidated fund that was directly targeted at the educational needs of minority ethnic children, in contrast with services provided under Section 11 that included a wide range of anti-discriminatory and anti-racist measures that extended beyond the sphere of education. The emphasis on the grant has been on promoting achievement among those minority ethnic groups who appear to be underperforming in schools. The grant is devolved to schools on the basis of the number of EAL (English as an Additional Language) pupils, the number of ethnic minorities and the number of pupils receiving free school meals.

A further funding mechanism was the Vulnerable Children Grant, the purpose of which was to 'support attendance, integration or reintegration into school...and to provide additional educational support to enable vulnerable children to achieve their potential'. Unlike the EMAG, which explicitly aimed to enhance school performance, there was scope within the Vulnerable Children Grant to adopt a holistic approach covering pastoral aspects of support. Asylum-seeker and refugee children were identified as one of seven groups eligible to receive this support.

The introduction of these new funding mechanisms did not allay concerns regarding the potentially deleterious impact of giving support to one group rather than another. Rutter condemns what she describes as 'central government structures and policy initiatives' that have 'widened the split between the education of refugees and minority ethnic communities' (Rutter, 2006, p125). Arnot and Pinson, in a 2005 report on asylum-seeker and refugee children's education, point to the government finding that where the EMAG had increasingly been used to meet the needs of asylum-seeker and refugee pupils, this gave 'less flexibility to focus on raising the achievement of British-born minority ethnic pupils' (Arnot and Pinson, 2005, p21).

These responses recall early anthropological formulations of the 'limited good' in which the

> desired things in life such as land, wealth, health, friendship and love...power and influence, security and safety, *exist in finite quantity* and are *always in short supply,* but in addition there is *no way directly...to increase the available quantities.* It follows from this that *'an individual or a family can improve a position only at the expense of others'.*
>
> (Foster, 1965, p296, emphasis in original)

The formulation was originally developed in relation to peasant communities, conceptualised as existing in a world very different to modern industrialised societies. However, it is arguable that it also has contemporary relevance in the present context. As formulated in the early work of Foster, a prerequisite for the development of what he refers to as the 'image of the limited good' is an existence in which there are considerable external constraints to the exercise of agency. This constraint is, of course, starkly evident in the distribution and maintenance of land and natural resources in traditional peasant economies. Indeed, as Scheper-Hughes has observed, Foster's formulation was deficient only inasmuch as it did not demonstrate how this 'image' was, in fact, 'an accurate assessment of the social reality in which most contemporary peasants live' (Scheper-Hughes, 1992, p548). With reference to the education of asylum seekers in the UK, evoking an image of the limited good may also be seen as a product of accurate assessment. Where there are only one or two funding resources available for specialised initiatives and services for such a disparate range of groups, it is not hard to see how the image of the 'limited good' can arise and result in a competitive orientation.

The problems and conflicts recorded by Rutter highlight the tensions that can arise when minority groups and their advocates are forced to compete for finite public resources. Longer established immigrant communities may have achieved a level of recognition and a degree of participation that has been fought hard and which they may see as being partially eroded by the incorporation of newer groups. Section 11 monies represented a limited good in this sense and the concerns surrounding the incorporation of refugees related not only to potential financial implications for projects associated with settled black and minority ethnic groups, but more broadly to a dilution of its purposes to incorporate needy white refugee groups.

Here the formulation of the limited good suggests an interrelationship between government agencies and minority ethnic groups and refugees, in this context as givers and receivers of resources. Within the educational sphere minority ethnic groups and refugees are routinely construed as having particular needs and, as such, requiring funding and forms of service provision beyond that found in mainstream services. The notion of special provision for particular groups extends well beyond the sphere of education and refugees and is both complex and controversial. Nancy Frazer has observed that in recent times, 'claims for the recognition of group difference have become increasingly salient...at times eclipsing claims for social equality' (Frazer, 1997, p2).

The notion of special provision in the British context is underpinned by a view of mainstream services as providing inadequately for particular groups. This perceived inadequacy is linked to evidence of the underachievement of specific groups in the educational system and also to more generalised views that groups have needs that are so specific and unique that mainstream services require special resources to cope with them.

Meso and micro level – local interpretation and implementation

As noted above, a meso level refers to the organisational configurations within which services are delivered and includes consideration of the interrelationship between various institutional 'actors' at a localised level. At this level it is particularly important to discern the extent to which provision in this area is 'top-down' and circumscribes the potential for the development of grassroots initiatives. The meso level is, I suggest, an analytically useful way of describing the processes whereby laws, guidelines and policies are interpreted and local initiatives developed. As defined here, this level of analysis is arguably most pertinent to what Esping-Anderson has defined as 'liberal' welfare regimes such as in the US, rather than more embedded 'conservative', such as in France or Germany or 'social democratic' regimes, such as characterise Scandinavian countries (Esping-Anderson, 1990).

From a social care perspective, the conservative and social democratic welfare regimes have arguably less diversity of provision and are more centrally managed through policy directives from central government (Goodwin, 1997). This may go some way towards explaining the diversity of 'bottom-up' initiatives in the UK as compared for example with the Netherlands and Sweden (Watters *et al.*, 2003). It also suggests potentially a more patchy, uneven and, at times, chaotic approach to social care within liberal regimes. However, it should also be noted that Esping-Anderson's regimes are 'ideal types' in the Weberian sense and that the overall position is rather fluid. For example, what Esping-Andersen identifies as conservative and social democratic countries have undergone significant shifts towards neoliberalism since the mid-1980s (Harvey, 2005).

Attention to a meso level consisting of approaches and initiatives at a local level is arguably most appropriate in contexts in which there are significant differences in the achievement of ethnic minorities. For example, within the UK girls and boys of Indian origin do significantly better in school than white girls and boys, while those of Bangladeshi or Pakistani origin generally do worse (IPPR, 2006; Schierup *et al.*, 2006). Within this context, models of 'racialised exclusion' based on nationally constructed comparative data do not engage with the complexities of varying results for particular ethnic groups and differences in regional and local contexts.

The importance of localised study is underlined in wide-ranging research examining community relations in the East End of London published in 2006. Here the authors noted that while Bangladeshi children's performance in national examinations remained below the national average, their performance improved significantly throughout the 1990s, with 46 per cent recording more than five GCSE passes between A to C in 2002 as compared to a national average of 51 per cent passes. This performance was above the average for the area and exceeded that for white children studied who achieved a pass rate of 30 per cent in 2002. The reasons behind this marked improvement were not without controversy, with some white parents claiming that Bangladeshi children received extra attention and support from teachers who were under pressure from national and local government to improve the performance of this group (Dench *et al.*, 2006, p142). Again, here the responses of white parents interviewed in the study suggests the salience of the concept of the 'limited good' in that they felt the resources of the system were no longer supportive of their children. Whatever the reasons behind the change, it is notable that positive results were achieved within a local context involving a group who were widely seen as having low levels of educational achievement. Interestingly, the authors note that one of the emerging challenges in schools in the area relates to the arrival of Eastern European asylum seekers with the result that, 'there is now an increasing number of *white* non-English speaking children in the schools' (ibid., p140, emphasis in original).

Arguably, a generalised formulation of racialised exclusion is most appropriate in contexts in which there is evidence of undifferentiated disadvantage experienced by migrants and new ethnic minorities with their background in non-OECD countries (Schierup *et al.*, 2006). The generalised exclusion of members of these groups suggests the importance of broad national strategies aimed at addressing widespread racial discrimination. However, where there is evidence of a complex situation in which certain groups of migrants and ethnic minorities are doing comparatively well while other groups are not, a more nuanced approach is suggested. Moreover, an advantage arising from allowing a level of flexibility at a local level is that initiatives can be developed that could be reproduced elsewhere. A glance across the landscape of service provision for refugees in the UK reveals a highly complex picture with a wide variety of central and local government initiatives, and a considerable engagement of a range of voluntary and community organisations. However, as noted earlier, the potential strengths of this diversity are often mitigated by a patchiness of provision in which good practice in one locality may be juxtaposed by very poor practice in another. This diversity is apparent in the sphere of education and results in a plethora of policies, strategies and initiatives.

In a wide-ranging study into local authority responses to the education of asylum-seeker and refugee children in England, Arnot and Pinson identified a range of distinctive policies and practices adopted in 58 areas. These included five distinctive types of policy responses towards meeting the educational needs of asylum-seeking children:

- specific category within a broader policy (28% of the sample)
- a comprehensive targeted policy (26% of the sample)
- language policy (16% of the sample)
- school guidance (16% of the sample)
- general policy in relation to special vulnerable groups (16% of the sample).

(Arnot and Pinson, 2005, p5)

The report highlights the complexity of the relationship between policy and practice. The authors argue that the absence of policy in some schools should not be taken to indicate an underdeveloped support system 'since some Local Education Authorities preferred not to develop explicit policies but focussed on provision' (ibid., p5). This implies that the evaluation of schools' performance should not presume that an absence of policy is tantamount to an absence of good services, as arrangements were made 'on the ground' often without explicit formulation. Furthermore, the differing approaches identified were offered within a broader funding context in which asylum seekers and refugees were largely invisible as 'there is no specific funding arrangement to support the education of asylum seeker and refugee children' (Arnot and Pinson, 2005, p5). This absence of specific funding was consistent with the view of Ofsted, the national schools' inspection body, that argued for 'the importance of addressing their needs through mainstream approaches to inclusion and racial equality' (ibid.).

From a broader perspective, the methodology adopted by Arnot and Pinson is reflective of the distinctive character of policy processes towards refugees in the UK. As in the case of a range of policy-oriented studies in the field, a typology of service responses is generated through an initial mapping of local policy and practices, and then may become a basis for the emergence of examples of good practice. To briefly give one of a number of possible examples of this approach, the UK Audit Commission, which has responsibility for ensuring the best use of public money, undertook a study of the support provided to asylum seekers in the UK in 2000 (Audit Commission, 2000). This followed the introduction of new dispersal and support arrangements for asylum seekers in the Immigration and Asylum Act of 1999. In generating recommendations, the authors went round the country identifying examples of 'good practice' that were described through a series of case studies. These were explicitly linked to the reports concluding recommendations. In methodological and practical terms, the approach is 'bottom up' in that the form of local policy and practice was, by no means, self-evident and could not be directly inferred from national directives. The complexity of the UK situation is revealed in a number of areas. Besides differences in policy, local authorities displayed differing educational models and concepts of good practice on the basis of which Arnot and Pinson proposed the following typology:

- EAL (English as an Additional Language) model
- holistic model
- minority ethnic model
- new arrivals model
- race equality model
- vulnerable children model.

(Arnot and Pinson, 2005, p6)

The authors point out that these models are not mutually exclusive and that several approaches may be present conterminously within a local education authority. They argue that the typology is important in that distinctive models 'suggest the logic that lies behind different practices and the support offered by a LEA or a school' (ibid., p41). The formulation of the models draws from the evidence gathered in the survey of local authorities, but offers a secondary and superimposed conceptual formation. As such, the proposed models may be seen as akin to the idea of 'ideal types' in the Weberian sense and may usefully serve a similar heuristic function in here exploring the responses of educational authorities to refugee children (Weber in Whimster, 2004, p388).

While the purpose of Arnot and Pinson's study appears to have been descriptive and analytical rather than evaluative, the authors do stress many of the positive features of the holistic model and it is appropriate to consider some of these in a little more detail here. They suggest that the model contains three specific areas of good practice: parental involvement, community links, and a multi-agency approach. Furthermore, it is identified as being underpinned with the following characteristics: the local education authority has experience with ethnic minority children, it promotes positive images of asylum-seeker and refugee pupils, it establishes clear indicators of successful integration, it has an ethos of inclusion and celebration of diversity, it has a holistic approach to provision and support and a caring ethos (ibid., p7). Using the areas of good practice identified by the authors, the following practical measures can be identified from the case studies they undertook:

Parental support and involvement

This aspect included the following:

- assistance in providing free school meals and free uniforms, providing each new arrival with a starter kit that included a school bag, notebooks and other essentials
- managing admissions based on an assessment of the needs of refugee families, including the need for the family to have a social network
- the appointment of cultural mediators whose role is to provide refugee children and parents with the opportunity to share their concerns with someone with the same language and culture; the cultural mediator's role includes providing advocacy for the families

- the running of training for staff on how to encourage parental involvement
- a weekly surgery to provide support to parents on issues relating to admissions
- the provision of multi-lingual information booklets, cassettes and DVDs for parents including information on the education system and the local education authority
- the development of a directory of services called 'parent aid' that drew on a systematic recording of issues raised by parents.

Community links

This aspect included the following:

- the maintenance of an active website that includes examples of good practice, information of relevance to refugees drawn from a range of government sources and examples of letters supporting families who are facing deportation
- a range of training and awareness raising initiatives directed at school staff, governors and community members, aimed towards encouraging a more empathic and informed understanding of the challenges facing asylum seekers and refugees
- developing educational programmes for refugee week aimed at engaging with pupils across schools.

Inter-agency work

This aspect included the following:

- the establishment of multi-agency consortia to identify and address the range of needs asylum seekers and refugees are faced with
- the appointment of 'advisory support' staff whose function is to advise schools on how best to support asylum-seeking and refugee pupils
- the development of local policies aimed at the social inclusion of asylum seekers and refugees that identifies the roles to be played by a variety of agencies.

The items identified above offer only a brief indication of the elements identified in Arnot and Pinson's 'holistic model' and readers are referred to the report for a full description. It is important to note that the model was identified as present in 18 out of 58 schools studied and the majority offered a considerably more limited approach to the children and their parents. This scenario is in turn symptomatic of the strengths and limitations of what may be referred to as the 'British' model, in that pockets of 'good practice' coexist with examples of relatively weak service provision. One particularly impressive feature of the holistic model described here is that it rests on a conceptualisation of the refugee child as located within a wider context that includes her parents, her community, the host society and the particular legal and social challenges children and families face. The approach recognises that a positive educational experience rests on a series of interconnected strands.

Cindy Mels and Ilse Derluyn encountered some similarities of approach in their preliminary investigation of schools' provision for refugee children in Belgium (2006). While their brief study focused particularly on the role of refugee parents in schools, they drew broader lessons regarding the essential features of a collaborative approach. Drawing on focus groups with refugee parents, the researchers found that parents were generally very positive about receiving home visits by representatives of the school. They regarded the appointment of intermediaries with responsibility for 'newcomer education' as a positive development and appreciated opportunities for discussion about their child's education. They were similarly positive about taking opportunities to engage in school activities, for example, after-school clubs, but often felt unable to join these owing to job commitments or looking after young children at home.

The parents were very highly motivated towards their children learning Dutch (the study was based in a Flemish region) and were worried that the high concentration of migrants in some schools may hinder the possibilities for learning the language. While generally quite positive about their role there was, interestingly, some concern expressed about the use of interpreters at meetings with teachers of the groups that this would not encourage the learning of Dutch. Mels and Derluyn found that while it was difficult for many parents to attend the focus groups, once there they became highly motivated and engaged. They were extremely keen to learn more about the school, the Belgian education system, social services and Belgian society in general and had numerous comments and suggestions as to how the school experience may be improved. These included more regular group discussions with parents, an expansion of the role of school intermediaries including more school visits, and increased numbers of Belgian children in the school to give their children more opportunity to learn Dutch.

I suggest that these examples and those derived from the work of Rutter, Arnot and Pinson, Dench *et al.* and numerous descriptive commentaries on policy and practice indicate both the importance of certain approaches on the meso level and a convergence of views as to what may constitute the key components of good practice. Firstly, and fundamentally, it is essential that there is the potential for development at the meso level. This requires a certain freeing up of funding and resources of local education authorities and schools to develop local policies and practices that are receptive to the needs and wants of refugee children and their parents. From this the possibility emerges of developing strategies involving liaison with local communities, home visits, parent–teacher liaison, provision of language support and after-school activities.

As outlined above, the micro level concerns the direct interface with refugee children and includes the development of special school programmes and activities delivered within the classroom. As a range of researchers have indicated, the provision of services range from total incorporation within the mainstream education system with little or no specialist support, to the positioning of refugee children within completely separate educational units. Intermediate models include the incorporation of refugees in schools with varying degrees of support and include the provision of special programmes designed to facilitate the integration of refugee children into the school and the wider society. The shape of these differing approaches is influenced directly by explicit educational policies formulated at a macro level and furthermore by broader policies relating to migrants and minority ethnic groups. The latter are in turn influenced by complex relationships between the media, politicians and the electorate and infused with what Schierup *et al.* have referred to as the 'political and cultural crisis and transformation of the nation and established national identities'. They argue that the most conspicuous manifestation of this crisis of the nation has been the upturn of new nationalist racist-populist political movements centred on the 'problem of immigration' (Schierup *et al.*, 2006, p3).

This crisis, crucially fuelled by events and the nature of reactions to 9/11, the London and Madrid bombings and the murder of the Dutch film-maker Theo van Gogh resulted in the strengthening of dichotomising discourses in which Muslims were construed as the 'other' and a potential threat to social cohesion. The events led to widespread questioning of policies towards migrants and ethnic minorities, particularly with respect to the adoption or continuation of multiculturalism. It is not appropriate here to explore these debates in detail, but it is important for the present purposes to note that these factors impinge on the micro level. In many countries these events and debates have resulted in a movement away from multi-culturalism towards 'integration' or 'assimilation' with a strong emphasis being placed, for example, on the responsibility of migrants to learn the host country's language and demonstrate allegiance to its purported norms and values. Somewhat paradoxically, within the UK this shift has coincided with a curtailing of free English language lessons for adult asylum seekers from 2007, leading children's charities to point to the deleterious impact this is likely to have on parental support and integration of asylum seeker's children (Ward, 2006).

These examples illustrate the interrelationship between educational provision for refugee children at a macro, meso and micro level. A multi-level analysis is important not only to provide broad analysis of the range of salient factors involved in the provision of educational programmes, but also at a practical level to identify the processes necessary for their implementation. These may also be considered as 'top-down' and 'bottom-up' factors in service development with the interplay between these aspects influenced in turn by the national construction of distinctive welfare regimes. A further dynamic, which will be considered in the following chapters, are processes of 'incorporation' and 'non-incorporation' of refugee children within services and how this relates to children occupying particular 'problem spaces'.

6   The role of special programmes

A common approach to meeting the needs of refugee children is through the establishment of special programmes. An investigation of the social care of refugee children reveals a wide range of such programmes; from initiatives in the educational sphere, to advocacy and counselling. Some are broadly based and seek to provide a comprehensive range of services, while others are targeted at very specific needs. In this chapter a range of special programmes are explored particularly in the education and mental health fields, with specific attention paid to the influential Pharos school programmes that originated in the Netherlands but have been incorporated into services for refugee children in a number of countries. These special programmes, while emerging in specific national contexts, are influenced by pervasive discourses on the problems of refugee children. Before examining the programmes and their philosophical underpinnings I outline some specific discourses and their impact on the locating of refugee children within specific 'problem spaces'.

Identifying the 'problems' of refugee children

Practices in the classroom, as in other contexts in which refugee children are positioned, are appropriately viewed as not detached, but as a microcosm of wider social and political currents. While discourses on assimilation and integration impinge on the teaching of refugee children, a range of discourses that are more specifically linked to refugee children powerfully influence teaching. These act as a framework or a lens through which refugee children are viewed as having particular needs for services to respond to. They are routinely embedded in policy directives that provide the context for working directly with refugee children and, at a micro level, represented by teachers within the school setting. As Popkewitz and Brennan argue in a significant contribution to educational theory,

> speech is ordered through principles of classification that are socially formed through a myriad of historical practices. When teachers talk about school as management, teaching as the production of learning, or children as being 'at-risk', these terms are not merely the personal words of the teacher, but are produced in the context of historically constructed 'ways of reasoning'.
>
> (Popkewitz and Brennan, 1997, p293)

In the case of refugee children, these historically constructed ways of reasoning include three particular and contemporary discursive domains, specifically those pertaining to *child development, trauma,* and *risk and resilience.* What I refer to here as discursive domains relates to what Foucault has referred to as 'dividing practices', whereby people are categorised and classified within distinctive technologies of governing. As Nikolas Rose has argued, 'childhood is the most intensively governed sector of personal existence' (Rose, 1999a, p123). Government of the child and in other areas is realisable through 'discursive mechanisms that represent the domain to be governed as an intelligible field with specifiable limits and particular characteristics' (Rose, 1999b, p33). The role of child development in providing a normative basis and evaluative criteria in studies of diverse groups of children has been discussed previously and I amplify these issues further here. I also examine discourses on trauma and risk and resilience as these routinely underpin a range of special programmes for refugee children.

As Aiwa Ong and others have suggested, the employment of specific discourses in relation to the social welfare of refugees is not a 'one-way street' in which practices are simply imposed on populations. She notes, on the basis of her fieldwork with Cambodian refugees in the US,

> the effects of the technologies of governing – as relayed through social programmes and experts seeking to shape one's subjectivity – can be rejected, modified, or transformed by individuals who somehow do not entirely come to imagine, to act, or to be enabled in quite the ways envisioned in the plans and projects of authorities.
>
> (Ong, 2003, p16)

At the micro level, Ong lists a series of mediators who translate the problematics of government into everyday operations referred to by Rose as 'experts of subjectivity' who 'transfigure existentialist questions...and the meaning of suffering into technical problems about the most effective ways of managing malfunction and improving the "quality of life"' (Rose quoted in Ong, 2003, p16). Within the present context, the discourses relating to refugee children embodied in a range of policies and practices, are predominant in a range of professional groups working with refugees including teachers, social workers and doctors.

A discourse on child development is not, of course, confined to refugee children but is ubiquitous in studies and professionalised practices relating to childhood. As indicated above, where it may be particularly salient with respect to refugee children is in processes whereby children's progress is measured against what are postulated as general norms. Western models of child development are heavily influenced by the work of seminal figures such as Freud, Piaget, Bowlby and Erikson who suggested distinctive models of development. Severe disruption from the chronological sequencing of development could result in aberrant behaviour and mental health problems. As noted in Chapter 2, these models were developed within specific Western contexts yet, in a variety of institutional settings, formed basic and universalised templates for the assessment of children with little or no regard for cultural differentiation. They help constitute what Nicola Ansell has referred to as the 'global model of childhood', which still infuses contemporary studies of refugee children with implicit normative statements regarding developmental stages (Ansell, 2005). For example, in a study into the psychological well-being of refugee children, Somali children in the West were described as having a differing pace of development, experiences of war 'had the effect of accelerating their development, the context of war having undoubtedly affected their developmental pathway' (Davies and Webb, 2000, p547). Boyden and de Berry argue by contrast that a concern with universalised norms of child development in research on children in war can have the effect of obscuring important issues relating to culture, social power and identity. They point towards more nuanced approaches that reach 'beyond the commonalities of the human condition to highlight also major individual differences between the young'. These arise through a combination of genetic heritage and personal agency and their interaction in 'a specific set of historical, social and cultural circumstances' (Boyden and de Berry, 2004, xvi).

Trauma

A discourse on trauma is prevalent in many of the scholarly articles and policy formulations on refugee children. It is by no means confined to the mental health literature and extends to general material on refugee children and work in the educational sphere. Indeed its ubiquity is such that one can be forgiven for assuming from the results of literature searches on refugee children that the word must have been inadvertently included in the search criteria. Rutter's observation from her own literature review on refugee children is that 76 per cent of the material comprised what she contends were 'psychological research monographs about trauma' (Rutter, 2006, p4).

At least three reasons may be identified for the prevalence of this discourse. First, it may be seen as linked to the emergence of post-traumatic stress disorder as an official psychiatric condition in the wake of the Vietnam War. The anthropologist Allan Young has examined the various social, economic and political factors that gave rise to the diagnosis, demonstrating that it was not simply the product of medical discovery (Young, 1995). As embedded in psychiatric nosology, it drew a direct clinical linkage between the effects of war, human rights violations, major ecological disturbances and the emergence of a specific psychiatric illness. Given that, by definition, refugees have escaped from a well founded fear of persecution and many would be victims of gross abuses of human rights, it is not difficult to see why a hypothesis developed that many were suffering from trauma and its after-effects. Diagnostic tools were subsequently developed and tested on refugees with varying results, many indicating high levels of post-traumatic stress disorder (PTSD).

A second possible reason relates to the ubiquity of a 'therapy culture' as identified by Furedi and others in which experiences that would once have been thought normal are being redefined as syndromes requiring medical intervention

(Furedi, 2003). Within the refugee field, Summerfield has drawn attention not only to the wide application of the trauma discourse to refugees but also to what he sees as the ideological motivations and financial interests that may underpin it (Summerfield, 1999). According to him, the ubiquity of the discourse internationally is symptomatic of a process of psychiatric imperialism that seeks to impose Western value systems, interests and treatments on populations in the developing world. In so doing, it undermines traditional models of solace and support and fails to engage with refugees in finding out about what they themselves might view as priorities. It may be, for example, that they feel their greatest medium-term priorities are education and employment and that the availability of these would do much to overcome natural feelings of suffering and despair.

A third reason is perhaps less suggestive of pernicious motivation and relates to processes of refugee recognition in industrialised countries and the strategic and tactical role of mental health workers and refugee advocates. I have referred to this previously as 'strategic categorisation' (Watters, 2001a). It draws on evidence of a shift in industrialised countries away from granting asylum seekers refugee status on the grounds of persecution, towards allowing them more limited rights to remain in potential host countries on humanitarian grounds. These include a shift in emphasis towards what Fassin has referred to as the 'suffering body' and legitimisation based on identification of health and mental health problems (Fassin, 2001). This represents a move away from the social and political towards the individual and the clinical.

Where strategic categorisation differs from Summerfield's broad critique is in the emphasis placed on the role of various health and social care professionals and representatives of civil society organisations in strategically and tactically operating within the wider system. As such, they are not necessarily mere functionaries operating within a hegemonic discourse, but actors who may engage strategically to further refugees' aspirations in sophisticated ways. The concept has, as such, complementarities with Lipsky's 'street level bureaucrats' who are aware of political and policy contexts but who operate within them in strategic ways (1980). Within the present context, the trauma discourse may be employed in a way that reflects awareness of systemic realities but is employed at micro and meso levels to seek the best possible outcomes for clients. As I have argued elsewhere, this should not been seen as a form of deception on the part of health workers, NGOs and refugee advocates, but rather a placement of emphasis on real and verifiable problems refugees are facing that are likely to engender the best practical outcomes (Watters, 2001a).

Arguably the potential for strategic categorisation is present to a higher degree within welfare systems where a significant role is played by a variety of actors from non-governmental bodies. The agencies mediate between the refugee and a range of statutory legal bodies and social and health care services and can provide expertise on particular cultural and clinical aspects. I refer here for example to agencies in industrialised countries such as the Bicultural Team in the Refugee Council and the Medical Foundation for the Care of Victims of Torture in London, STARTTS in Sydney, Maison d'Amite in Montreal and the Platform for the Reception of Unaccompanied Minors in Paris (Red Cross, 2006). These agencies occupy intermediate positions between refugees and statutory institutions and incorporate a counsellor/advocate role into their services whereby, besides providing direct services, they also help refugees to locate the most appropriate individuals and agencies to support them. In some instances they provide specialist support in clinical assessment and evidence of torture and provide expertise in legal hearings.

The agencies are far from the rather supine and complicit image of the bi-cultural worker in Ong's study of the mental health care of Cambodians in San Francisco, as they frequently challenge institutional practices on behalf of their clients (Ong, 2003). This is not to imply that they are not working within environments in which they face considerable constraints. The agencies are normally embedded within institutional policies and procedures conforming to legally constituted requirements. Others may operate as charities but undertake work with refugees through highly prescriptive contracts drawn up by government agencies. However, as Evans and Harris have argued in their study of social work and street level bureaucracy, 'a proliferation of rules and regulations should not automatically be equated with greater control over professional discretion; paradoxically, more rules may create more discretion'. They note, for example, situations where management rules may actually be an impediment to the supervision of their work, 'rules often collapse complex goals, which have many, often conflicting or outright contradictory, aspects (Evans and Harris, 2004, p879). Evans and Harris offer astute observations of the environments in which many social care professionals operate. However, my suggestion here is a little broader and concerns not only individual professionals but also agencies that operate in ways that implicitly or explicitly challenge policy. They often do so not only by challenging rules but also by drawing on rules and policies linked to different domains that have a bearing on the client's welfare and may challenge what I have referred to as an immigration trajectory. Thus laws and policies relating to aspects of child welfare or human rights or local authority policies on destitution or housing may be invoked strategically. Despite its ubiquity it is important therefore not simply to locate trauma within a homogenising discourse on refugees, but to recognise both that trauma symptoms are present within a proportion of the refugee population and that this fact may be emphasised strategically by a range of professionals and advocates concerned for refugees' welfare.

Risk and resilience

Resilience has been authoritatively defined in psychological literature as 'a dynamic developmental process reflecting evidence of positive adaptation despite significant life adversity' (Cicchetti, 2003, pxx). Over the past three decades there have been numerous studies of children and resilience, focusing for example on poverty and urban deprivation, children exposed to violence, and parental abuse and separation (see Luthar, 2003). Researchers have described resilience as 'an inference about a person's life that requires *two fundamental judgements* 1) that the person is "doing okay", and 2) that there is now or has been significant risk or adversity to overcome' (Masten and Powell, 2003, p4, emphasis in original). Put simply, the concept of resilience challenges assumptions of a straightforward and deterministic relationship between the experience of adversity and developmental outcomes. Michael Rutter developed the concept of protective factors that act to mediate the effects of exposure to adversity and proposed an interactive relationship between the protective factor, the risk exposure, and the outcome (Ferguson and Horwood, 2003, p131). Resilience has also been the subject of a number of longitudinal studies in which a variety of potential risk factors have been identified including, for example, the relationship between psychiatric risk and severe marital distress, low socio-economic status, large family size or overcrowding, paternal criminality, maternal psychiatric disorder and placement of a child in foster care (Luthar, 2003).

The cumulative deleterious potential of risk factors is reflected in policy formulations and academic studies in which refugee children are often characterised as assailed by multiple risks. In a review of interventions for refugee children in New Zealand schools, published in 2006 by the New Zealand Ministry of Education, refugee children are described as potentially '"at risk" even without the additional risks associated with being a refugee' (Hamilton *et al.*, 2006, p30). The risk factors of being a refugee are enumerated; experience of war, famine, persecution, violence, flight, loss of home, family, friends, a way of life and involuntary migration. Furthermore, resilience factors at home may turn into risk factors in the host nation. For example, having parents with high educational qualifications is normally a positive factor, but if these parents are unable to have their qualifications recognised and cannot find employment, this may be a risk factor (ibid., p32).

From a Foucauldian perspective, Rose argues that the emphasis on risk represents a fundamental shift from viewing pathology residing in the individual to 'a combination of factors that are not necessarily pathological in themselves'. These are the subjects of expert interventions aimed at 'identifying, recording, assessing risk factors in order to predict future pathology and take action to prevent it' (Rose, 1998, p94). The association of multiple risk factors with refugee children encourages professionals to view them as highly vulnerable, and institutions to place them automatically in contexts where they receive special provisions. While references to resilience occur in a great deal of the policy documents and guidelines relating to refugee children, I go along with Rutter's assertion that a good deal of the references are somewhat 'tokenistic'. They appear as an explicit or implicit acknowledgement of the potency of the various research findings and critiques by, for example, Summerfield (1999), Eastmond (1998) or Muecke (1992), who point to the way in which refugees are pathologised in research and service provision. Muecke, for example, has suggested that rather than focusing on refugee pathology, a new paradigm should emerge in which refugees are seen instead as prototypes of resilience despite major losses and stressors (Muecke, 1992). However, despite these influential critiques, references to resilience are often embedded in policy documents that are oriented primarily towards advising professionals of the numerous risks and vulnerabilities associated with refugee children.

Much work on the resilience of refugee children is 'ecological' in orientation and focuses on the potential impact of factors in the environment surrounding the children, such as family relationships, communities and institutions, including schools. As such it has often close complementarities with the social capital literature. In other words, the environment is viewed through a lens of numerous potential threats or supports to the child's well-being. Those community resources that are viewed as supporting resilience include good schools, connections to 'prosocial' organisations such as clubs or religious groups, the quality of the neighbourhood through public safety, collective supervision, the presence of libraries and recreation centres and good quality health and social care (Masden and Powell, 2003, p13). These formulations however may give little indication of the ecological factors that can influence resilience in refugee children. A school may be 'good' in that it is well equipped and achieves a high educational standard, but that may tell us little about the experiences refugee children have in it. They may be singled out by students and teachers as a special group and be subjected to discrimination and bullying. Good community centres, health and social care services may actually increase refugees' feelings of vulnerability and isolation if they feel excluded from them. Furthermore, the responses of community members can, it is argued, itself be a risk factor in that, following the symbolic interactionists, 'we are who we think others think we are', and, in this way, members of minority groups may internalise negative images (Szalacha *et al.*, 2003, p421).

Psychoanalytically oriented studies of refugee children's resilience address the emotional and cognitive qualities resilient children develop. For example, drawing on in-depth studies of Israeli and Palestinian children, Apfel and Simon argue that characteristics that contribute to resiliency include resourcefulness, curiosity and intellectual mastery, the ability to conceptualise and generate knowledge, flexibility in emotional experience, access to autobiographical memory, having a goal for which to live, a need and ability to help others and a vision of a moral order (Apfel and Simon, 2000, p126). They argue that the presence of these qualities is dependent on the interactions children have with adults around them and with other children. In their list of qualities and attributes, the authors note the particular role of images of good and sustaining figures, usually parents, 'even if these images might at times be critical and demanding as well as warm, loving and encouraging'. The authors also strongly invoke the importance of 'a sense of activity rather than passivity'.

While here there is limited engagement with a consideration of the interrelationship between institutions and the affective and cognitive capacities of refugee children, the study does suggest questions regarding the extent to which the regimes of care that refugee children receive may actually undermine the development of resilience. If, as is contended in many studies, resilience is closely linked to a sense of agency and empowerment, then asylum regimes that place refugee children and their families in positions where they are unable to make decisions and exercise choices are likely to erode the potential to develop resilience. In other words, in situations where asylum seekers are placed in highly institutionalised settings where they are 'provided for' in terms of their basic needs but not allowed to influence aspects of their environment, vulnerability is likely to increase.

There are several recent examples that indicate the importance of refugees' agency in promoting resilience. In one, Maja Korac undertook a comparative qualitative study into the resettlement experiences of refugees in the Netherlands and Italy. In the Netherlands, there was a high level of systematic government control over the processes asylum seekers and refugees went through in responding to their claims and in managing their accommodation and welfare. In Italy, there was a far less systematic approach, with many left almost to fend for themselves through surviving on the streets. Despite the hardships they had to endure, Korac contends that her results showed that refugees felt they were in a preferable situation in Italy as they had some control over their lives. On the basis of her findings, Korac argues that countries should 'acknowledge refugees as social actors rather than turning them into policy objects in order to facilitate integration' (Korac, 2003, p51).

In another study focusing on Iranian women refugees, Ghorashi similarly emphasises the disempowering environment for refugees in Dutch society, particularly in the light of recent policies:

> Dutch asylum policies that went into effect in the 1990s influenced newly arriving asylum seekers by preventing them from participating in society. They also affected ex-refugees by creating an image of the refugee as helpless and victimized. The new regulations, which isolate refugees and make them state dependents, provide those proponents of exclusive discourses with the justification they need to picture refugees as 'the problems' of the society.
>
> (Ghorashi, 2005)

On the basis of her interviews with the Iranian women, she noted that refugees drew a direct correlation between the post-migration environment and the mental and emotional problems that had accompanied their flight:

> Not having a chance to build a new life makes it impossible to gain distance from the past by becoming active participants in the new society. Asylum seekers do not have the chance to deal with their feelings of guilt, and as a result this feeling grows day by day. They feel powerless. 'All we do is eat and sleep; we live like animals' [...] 'Each day is the same, every day I know what will happen, it's killing me'.
>
> (ibid., p190)

It is interesting to note that building a new life was viewed as the critical factor in overcoming the tribulations of the past. It offered the chance to create some psychological and emotional distance from what had gone before. Being placed in institutional settings with no control over their lives was viewed as seriously exacerbating their problems. These experiences accord with more general evidence linking the deterioration in mental health of asylum seekers in industrialised countries with immigration and asylum procedures. Silove and colleagues, for example, in a number of studies, have demonstrated strong correlation between specified aspects of asylum procedures in Australia and declining mental health. This link is demonstrated in a wider review of evidence from industrialised countries of the impact of post-migration factors and mental health (Silove *et al.*, 2000).

Docile bodies? Devitalisation and the refugee child

Issues of risk and vulnerability in post-migration environments have come to the fore in a dramatic fashion in Sweden in relation to a phenomenon variously described as 'devitalisation' or 'severe withdrawal'. In 2005, Swedish authorities recorded that a total of 424 children from asylum-seeking families were suffering from a condition they referred to as 'severe withdrawal behaviour'. Salient characteristics were food refusal and weight loss, social withdrawal, and partial or complete refusal to move, speak or attend to self-care. While similar cases had been recorded in other countries, these had been linked to quite different social circumstances and were largely associated with girls who were thought to have suffered sexual abuse. The Swedish cases were the first and, at the time of writing, the only large-scale manifestation of this problem among refugee children. Swedish investigators sought to establish evidence among asylum seekers in other European countries but could find little or none, even from within other Nordic countries. Other unique features of the Swedish situation were the prevalence of the condition in roughly equal numbers among both boys and girls and its presence both in very young children under the age of eight and in older children in their late teens. Furthermore, there were differences in the family dynamics between the Swedish and other cases in that in Sweden it appeared not to originate in family problems and parents tried to help the child as far as they could. Also, the children tended to be surrounded by other members of an extended family (Hessle, 2005).

The matter gave rise to considerable consternation within Swedish authorities and in the population at large, with the modus operandi through which the phenomenon was investigated reflecting the polarities in perspective. For some, the phenomenon was reflective of the processes of disempowerment inherent in the Swedish asylum system, while others thought it was part of a cynical ploy initiated by the parents of the children to further their asylum applications. The government appointed a national co-ordinator to investigate the matter and issue in-depth reports on the prevalence of the phenomenon, develop methods for dealing with children at risk, and initiate preventive action. The role also included the encouragement of new methods of co-operation and the promotion of exchange and knowledge in the field.

One finding concerned the origins of the children and showed that as many as 85 per cent whose country of origin was known came from the former Soviet Union (53%) and former Yugoslavia (31.4%). Some 26.7 per cent of those for whom there was data on ethnic origin came from 'two particularly vulnerable minority groups in central Asia and Kosovo' (Hessle, 2005, p30). The cultural characteristics of the groups were investigated and representatives from the various states of origin attended a conference in 2006 designed to gain a better understanding of the phenomenon. One of these delegates suggested that the families should be sent back to their country of origin and treated, while another suggested that the Swedish authorities were treating them too well.

It would be presumptuous and foolhardy to venture solutions in these brief pages to a phenomenon that has exercised the minds of numerous Swedish experts. The comments I make are more sociological and philosophical than clinical. As discussed previously, Fassin has noted a marked correlation in recent times between a decline in rates of those being granted asylum on the grounds of persecution and a concomitant increase in those being allowed to stay on humanitarian grounds. The latter phenomenon, Fassin noted, was particularly linked to reasons of ill health or what may be termed the legitimacy of the 'suffering body'. Thus the process may be described in Foucauldian terms as 'bio-legitimacy' (Fassin, 2001). To use a concept I have employed elsewhere, being sick represents an *avenue of access* through which people may earn a right to stay. Evidence of possible pathology gives rise to an institutional shift from the reception centre to the hospital and the outpatient clinic, from what I have broadly described as the immigration to the welfare trajectory.

Official reports stress the weakness of many of the families' claims for asylum and the fact that they may have had a history of having claims rejected. A significant number of the children have received residence permits following initial refusal of entry by the Swedish Migration Board. These decisions appear to directly relate to the children's condition. While they are generally viewed sympathetically, the parents of the children are subjected to thinly veiled criticism. According to one official report, 'there are a large percentage of parents who are insufficient, gravely mentally stressed or incapable of looking after their children, giving them hope or supporting them' (Hessle, 2005, p47). To continue the use of Foucauldian terminology, what we may be said to be witnessing is an extension of bio-legitimacy to the refugee child, linked to the simultaneous emergence and constriction of avenues of access.

A further conceptual formulation may be appropriate here. De Certeau has drawn a useful distinction between 'strategies' and 'tactics' and this distinction has been employed in anthropological writings on the theme of resilience (Scheper-Hughes, 1992). According to de Certeau, 'strategies are able to produce, tabulate, and impose', while tactics operate within predefined spaces and 'can only use, manipulate, and divert these spaces'. He identifies a process of production that can operate even within the most confined and totalitarian spaces, 'the child still scrawls and daubs on his schoolbooks; even if he is punished for this crime, he has made a space for himself and signs his existence as an author on it' (de Certeau, 1984, p31). The child's signing of existence has been noted earlier on the walls of the reception area in the port of Zeebrugge. In the present context the space for 'production' may ironically be confined to a practice of non-existence within a context in which there appears no prospect for an alternative exercise of agency.

Special programmes for refugee children

A common response towards meeting the health, social care and educational needs of refugee children is to establish special programmes for them. In countries experiencing a considerable influx of refugees, these are normally established through the work of UN agencies and a range of international NGOs. UNHCR records no less than 647 NGOs working with it as implementing partners on a range of programmes in 2006 (UNHCR, 2006c). In industrialised countries, programmes are often provided through charities and NGOs with specific funding from charitable institutions such as Save the Children, local or central government or international bodies such as the European Commission. The response to refugee children in industrialised countries is notable for the wide-ranging role played by these services in meeting the gaps that often occur in statutory provision. Within Europe, the Red Cross have documented some 40 examples of special programmes that offer good practice health care aspects of asylum reception (2006). While special programmes all have distinctive characteristics in terms of their internal organisation and modes of service provision, they do have certain structural features in common. These may be summarised in terms of a number of specific opportunities and constraints:

*   opportunities
    *   flexible working
    *   interagency collaboration
    *   task orientation/Innovation
*   constraints
    *   short-term duration
    *   insecure funding
    *   marginal status.

One advantage associated with special programmes is that they present an opportunity to work in a flexible way outside of the normal parameters of professional practice. They thus provide contexts in which roles can be blurred between the entrenched positions of, say, 'social worker' or 'counsellor' and workers can combine disciplinary approaches. This flexibility is particularly useful in contexts of shifting laws and policies and with client groups who may be moved between locations and institutions. Working flexibly provides an opportunity to be genuinely receptive to needs and develop approaches that take as a starting point the present problems facing a client. These can include accommodation, legal advice, health problems, isolation and family reunification. A special programme is unlikely to be able to meet all of these needs, but may have the flexibility to work with other agencies to arrange an effective response. In terms of organisational theory the approach may be described as 'task centred' with the characteristics of clear objectives and rather informal and egalitarian organisational structure (Handy, 1994).

While offering a context for 'getting things done' in a flexible and responsive way, special programmes do however typically operate within severe constraints.

They are typically funded for a limited period of time and face ongoing uncertainties concerning their long term viability. This has an impact on many aspects of the programmes' activities, including the recruitment and retention of staff. If a programme is, say, funded for three years, several months may be spent in recruiting staff and supporting them to work in the field before they are fully functional. Within a relatively short period of time they will have to consider their own longer term future and start to consider alternative positions. Besides its potential impact on staff morale, the short-term nature of projects can have a significant impact on clients. The programme may play a vital role in the lives of refugees, providing a central organising focus in a life full of uncertainties and anxiety. The prospect of its non-continuance may be extremely disturbing for clients and be a cause for losing trust in wider processes within a host society (Watters, 1996a). Inextricably linked to the short-term nature of special programmes is the often complex and time-limited financial arrangements on which they are based. These may include distinct funding from a number of sources such as international NGOs, national governments and transnational bodies such as the European Commission. Funders may have contributed to distinctive aspects of the programme and have specific requirements in terms of financial monitoring and programme evaluation. A final constraint relates to the marginal status of special programmes. They often exist at 'arm's length' from mainstream services and their distinctive modes of working make it difficult to incorporate them when funding sources are no longer available. Besides being marginal, they often have a low status in relation to professionals within mainstream organisations and can exert limited influence in promoting substantial and longer-term changes in policy and practice.

Despite these limitations, there are steps that can be taken to seek to ensure that special programmes do have longer-term impact. Funding bodies often insist on agreeing a strategy for encouraging the sustainability of programmes before approving funding. These are likely to include at least the production of a report on the programmes' activities and dissemination of lessons from the programme to a wide range of relevant organisations. In practice it is often difficult to assess the impact of programmes from these measures and reports often do not link to the formulation of broader strategies towards clients. The results of evaluations often do not appear to directly relate to decisions about the long-term future of programmes for refugees. Rather, their impact tends to be more diffuse and long term, contributing to a wider knowledge base on services and their impact. The following factors can contribute to the longer term sustainability of special programmes:

- prior agreement of criteria for continuation
- steering group
- links to policy processes.

One factor that is likely to have a significant influence on sustainability is the formulation of explicit criteria for the continuation of a programme at its very earliest stages. This would of course need to include contributions and agreements from appropriate funding organisations and mainstream services where the latter are expected to ensure the continuation of services. Sustainability is also likely to be influenced through the establishment of a steering group that oversees the general direction of the special programmes' work. The membership of these groups is important as this can influence positively the potential for the lessons emerging from the programme being introduced more widely into services. It also provides the potential for engaging with actual and potential funders during the life of the programme. More broadly, where feasible it is useful for special programmes to consider strategically their potentially wider role in the formulation of policy towards refugees through employing models of policy processes including ways in which the work of the programme may influence agenda settling (Kingdon, 1984).

While, from a practical perspective, these approaches may be helpful in sustaining programmes, a consideration of special programmes gives rise to broader questions regarding social responses to refugees. The gaps that special programmes often try to fill reflect the 'state of exception' that governs wider responses to refugees. Rather than eliciting the development of properly funded services that are supported by mainstream institutions, they are too often the subjects of *ad hoc* measures. Those working within special programmes are themselves often marginalised through working with these client groups, and enjoy little support. In the context of these constraints, where wider institutional support is provided to special programmes, this tends to be in accordance with services that are accommodated within prevailing discourses locating the problems of refugees and refugee children.

A discourse centred on risks and vulnerability underpins a range of special programmes that have been established for refugee children in both industrialised and non-industrialised countries. These emerge in a wide variety of locations where refugee children are present including schools, community centres and in a range of contexts within refugee camps. Jo de Berry and her colleagues have suggested two frameworks that guide programmes for children affected by war: the trauma approach and the psychosocial approach. They note that the former has been used for children in Rwanda, East Timor and Bosnia, while the psychosocial approach has been used in Palestine, Sri Lanka, Angola, Sierra Leone, East Timor and Bosnia. The authors have defined the characteristics of the frameworks in Table 6.1.

These frameworks can also be identified in a range of responses to refugee children in industrialised countries although they are unlikely to be as sharply delineated as suggested here. While what may be described as psychosocial approaches are found in a variety of settings, it is questionable, for example, whether these engage with children within family or community contexts or with their own subjectively defined priorities. It may be helpful here to explore the characteristics of special programmes for refugee children with reference to one influential example before considering further their wider role and implications.

Table 6.1

Focus	Main features
Trauma approach	
• Impact of war on children's mental health • Individual children	• Needs assessment is based on psychological and psychiatric measurements of post-traumatic stress disorder • Intervention consists of individual children receiving psychological and psychiatric treatment • Intervention makes the assumption that children can only be healed through technical assistance • Generally applicable for minority of war-affected children • High cost and dependent on technical expertise
Psychosocial approach	
• Impact of a range of problems on children's social relationships and emotional well-being • Groups of children in the context of their families and communities	• Needs assessment is based on subjective priorities defined by children and adults • Wide range of possible interventions, often community-based and involving children's groups. Focus on building children's relationships, re-establishing a sense of normality, supporting family life and giving children opportunities for emotional expression • Intervention based on identifying and strengthening children's own coping and resilience resources • Applicable for all war-affected children • Low cost and aims for local level sustainability

Adapted from de Berry *et al.*, 2003

The Pharos school programmes

The Pharos school prevention programmes for refugee children have grown steadily in influence since their introduction in the Netherlands from the mid-1990s to their wider use in a range of industrialised countries in 2007. Their dissemination has been supported by the enthusiastic response of a range of educational and child welfare agencies and by institutional backing from local and national educational authorities and the European Commission. Support from the latter has included an international project financed by the European Refugee Fund until 2006 aimed at disseminating two of the Pharos school programmes to six other European countries – Sweden, Italy, Germany, Austria, the UK and Ireland.

The programmes were developed by Pharos, defined on its website as the

> Dutch national refugee and health knowledge centre that concentrates on developing, studying and conveying knowledge – always practically applicable – in the field of health and health care for refugees. Pharos develops knowledge and methods for mental health care, medical care for asylum seekers, primary health care and youth services.
>
> (Pharos, 2007)

The organisation provides what may be defined as a consultancy role to national and local government in the field of refugees and health, rather than one of direct service provision. They produce programmes and methods that are subsequently purchased by those responsible for the direct provision of services.

The school prevention programmes have been described in detail in a substantial manual produced by de Ruuk as part of a wider study of the mental health and social care of refugees in Europe and the possibilities for transferring 'good practice' from one European country to another (de Ruuk, 2002; Watters *et al.*, 2003). A briefer description and discussion of the programmes is contained in a subsequent publication (Ingleby and Watters, 2002). An important feature of the programmes is that they are offered within the broader context of educational provision within refugee reception arrangements in the Netherlands. As noted, this is a context in which children are normally educated in reception centres where asylum seekers are based or in 'international bridge classes' where they spend between six months and three years before being transferred to mainstream classes. As a consequence, the programmes are targeted at groups of refugee children within relatively isolated contexts and do not involve interaction with children from the host society. A further feature is that Dutch teachers in partnership with local mental health services deliver the programmes.

The explicit philosophy underlying the programmes is that 'refugee children are normal children with sometimes extreme experiences' (de Ruuk, 2002, p32). They are underpinned by a view of refugee children's lives as consisting of a series of highly stressful events mapped onto a chronological sequence of pre-flight, flight, post-flight, arrival and screening, and the problems of acculturation and marginalisation following receiving permission to stay. Three potential protective factors; positive personality characteristics, a supporting family and an external social support system may mitigate these stressors. According to de Ruuk, the positive personality characteristics of the child include competence, coping behaviour and ego resilience. The development of competence is here described as following the work of Caplan on preventative psychiatry in which it is seen as the ability to effect changes in the environment. 'By strengthening the competence of the child, its coping skills can be improved, thereby preventing or reducing social and emotional problems. This is the main idea behind the Pharos school prevention programmes, especially those for primary school children' (de Ruuk, 2002, p15).

De Ruuk describes the programmes as being based on a model of three types of competence, *affective competence* derived from self-image and self-confidence, *social or behavioural competence* derived from social skills and social behaviour and *cognitive competence* linked to problem solving and learning skills. As such it appears to follow the models of competence suggested by Caplan and Weissberg and others (Caplan and Weissberg, 1988; Bloom, 1990).

Pharos has supported the development of knowledge in the field by in-house publications that elaborate on the relevance of psychological theories to refugees. In one, de Vries suggests that refugees can develop new coping strategies to defend against circumstances in which these have previously been 'unlearned' or forgotten in traumatic circumstances. Coping can also be undermined owing to the lack of control refugees experience during lengthy stays in reception centres (de Vries 2000, cited in de Ruuk, 2002). The development of ego resilience is here viewed as influenced by the care and attention of parents and through having enough 'structure' in their upbringing. Children who lack these will be psychologically more vulnerable (ibid.). More broadly, family support is recognised in the Pharos literature as being an especially important protective factor for refugee children but, at the same time, one that is often not working well.

Indeed the literature is sharply critical of some parents, 'workers in reception centres have seen parents leaving their children to fend for themselves, or parents who are not setting any boundaries. Sometimes mistreatment or abuse is seen' (ibid.). Elsewhere in the manual the effects of parents' mental health problems on children are highlighted, 'when the parents have psychological or psychiatric complaints, it can be said that the protective factor of "family" in many cases becomes just the opposite: a risk factor' (ibid., p20). Again it is asserted that,

> As a consequence of violence and acculturation, problematic situations within the family are frequently reported. Loss of autonomy, change of culture, change of role pattern and change of socio-economic status are stressors found in refugee families. Parents may have severe stress reactions and may be less capable of supporting their children.
>
> (Ibid.)

The view of the potential inadequacy and negative impact of parents on refugee children's mental health echoes those found in the Swedish reports on severe withdrawal behaviour referred to above.

In the Pharos manual, social support is differentiated in terms of support directed at the person and support directed at the situation, as follows.

Directed at the person

- emotional support – expressing respect, love, empathy, solidarity, physical affection, comfort and understanding

- appreciative support – expressing appreciation and acknowledgement, giving trust
- cognitive support – giving advice, information, explanation and feedback
- normative support – laying down behavioural standards, showing tolerance.

Directed at the situation

- material support – all forms of material help, like providing housing, money, transport etc.
- practical support – concrete practical help, like helping in the care (sic), or just having a fun time
- support for means of power and influence in social situations – mediating, for example in the asylum procedure to reduce stressors (de Ruuk, 2002, p16).

School is viewed in this context as a particularly important potential source of external support:

> School particularly functions as an important external support system for refugee children, because this is the place where new friends are made, where the child can play, actually be a child and have fun. School offers safety and structure. At school new customs, standards and values are learned, which help the child to feel more confident in its new environment. Above all it makes the child look ahead, instead of to the past. The school cannot replace the supporting role of parents, but it may compensate there (sic) where the parents lack in giving support.
>
> (van Aspern and Baan, 1998, cited in de Ruuk, 2002, p20)

Perspectives that highlight the ways in which refugee children may deviate from normal developmental trajectories further underpin the programmes. For example, the manual highlights the way in which the important developmental role of attachment as outlined in Bowlby's theories may be undermined: 'if attachment does not take place safely...the development of the child may be negatively influenced'. A unified view of the 'refugee experience' further underpins the specific difficulties of refugee adolescents. According to Pharos reports produced by Van der Veer (1998) and Tuk (1997), the adolescence of refugees is strongly influenced by the experiences preceding, during and after flight.

> In a stage of life in which one normally needs protection, clear boundaries, understanding and space for experimenting, these refugee children experience the opposite: violence and lawlessness are commonly seen. Furthermore the decision to flee is often made *for* them not by them.
>
> (Tuk, 1997, cited in de Ruuk, 2002, p20, emphasis in original)

Ten developmental 'tasks' are identified in the programmes to mitigate the effects of refugee children's experiences:

> taking better care of oneself, moving more independently through society, giving direction and substance to life autonomously, making and maintaining friendships with people from the peer group, integration of increasing sexual impulses, handling one's own aggressive impulses and aggression in the environment, reshaping the relationship with the parents, forming a perspective on the future, breaking through the isolation and coping with oneself and possible post-traumatic complaints.
>
> (ibid., p23)

These developmental tasks are proposed as a fundamental reorientation for refugee children in which social and cultural norms are substantially adapted or abandoned. The child has to adapt to a social order in which there is emphasis on autonomous action and individuality manifest in a range of spheres including friendships and sexuality. The cultures of the refugee children are viewed as contexts in which norms and values relating to family life, aggression and sexuality may have been developed that are not compatible with Dutch society. They are also viewed as imbuing refugee children with views and expectations of the future that are sometimes unrealistic. Their hopes may be too high, 'for example, in the case of poorly educated youngsters that think they can become a doctor or a pilot' (ibid., p23).

The programme literature identifies two fundamental preventative strategies for addressing the impact of the stressful experiences of refugee children: 1) strengthening the protective factors within the child by strengthening their 'competence' (as described above) and 2) strengthening the protective factor 'social support' by strengthening the competence of teachers who are supporting the children. Schools are viewed as uniquely suitable contexts for implementing these preventative approaches and holding the potential for the development of 'healing'. It is not overstating the matter to suggest that here they are seen as having little less than a soteriological function. According to the Pharos manual, 'school offers a safe, benevolent atmosphere, where the children have intensive contact with grown ups who are not a perpetrator or a victim. Teachers offer them a new identification model: they guarantee safety and function as guides in a new society'. Furthermore, school offers an environment where 'refugee children can recover their disturbed balance in a natural way' (ibid., p27).

These orientations and concerns underpinned the development of a total of seven school programmes that have been at various stages of evolution since approximately the mid-1990s. As noted above, particular programmes have been introduced into at least six other European countries and translated into a range of languages including English, German, Italian and Swedish. Four of the programmes are targeted at refugee children in primary education and three at those in secondary education. Two of the programmes are aimed at teachers working with refugees, one for those in primary education entitled, 'School as a Healer' and one for those working in secondary education entitled 'Refugee Youth at School'. The other five programmes are:

- Primary
    - The World United
    - Just Show Who You Are
    - Applause for Yourself
- Secondary
    - Refugee Lesson
    - Welcome to School

An outline of the content of the Pharos schools programmes

The World United, formally called FC the World was the first Pharos programme developed for primary schools and has been widely disseminated nationally and internationally. The aims of the programme are totally compatible with the orientations described above – to strengthen the affective, cognitive and social competence of the children plus additionally 'diminishing problematic behaviour like acting-out, socially anxious behaviour and learning problems'. A further and related explicit aim is to help children integrate their pasts with the present and the future (van Asperen and Baan, cited in de Ruuk, 2002, p35). Teachers working on the programme support children to tell their stories. The initiators of the programme have explained that in primary education little attention is given to the extraordinary background and experiences of these children. However, 'homesickness, memories of war, violence or the flight are common aspects of a refugee child's life and should not be neglected. Out of fear of being made fun of, these children often do not talk about their feelings' (ibid.). The programme was completed and published by Pharos in 1998 and later augmented by the School as a Healer training programme for teachers working with refugees and by Just Show Who You Are. The latter was designed for children who were relatively new to the Netherlands and did not have the verbal skills to participate in The World United. It consists of eight weekly lessons using primarily non-verbal methods.

It is targeted at children aged between 10 and 12 years old and the sessions focus on the following: me, my school, my home, my family, celebrating days, friendship, play and games and 'me, and you and we'. The sessions last between 75 and 100 minutes in which 'the children can talk about their experiences in the past and the present and their ideas about the future' (ibid., p37). They are supervised by two teachers, one who leads the session and one who plays an observer role. During the sessions the children make their own ME-book in which they can write about themselves and in which the products they have made during the sessions are collected. De Ruuk describes the initial session as follows:

> In the first lesson the children occupy centre stage: they tell each other about their background. The lesson starts with singing the first two stanzas of the FC the World song. Then a world map is shown, on which the children have to point out where they come from. A discussion about distances, national

flags and ways of coming to the Netherlands starts. Next, a game is played, in which one child has to tell the name and positive characteristics of another child. Goal of this game is to practice the giving and receiving of positive reactions in favour of their self image. The lesson is ended by introducing the Me-book, in which the children are asked to draw a self portrait.

(de Ruuk, 2002, p37)

As the weeks progress, the topics build in intensity with subjects such as 'where I live' and 'family' sometimes evoking the telling of stories of hardships and loss such as houses being destroyed or arriving in the Netherlands to find a father they hadn't seen for years with a new wife and the child with new brothers and sisters. The sessions begin and end with group singing of a communal song in which they celebrate being part of the same world.

While not explicitly formulated in these terms, the orientation of the programme is strongly individualistic and autobiographical. The children are guided towards giving cohesive accounts of themselves in which past, present and future is integrated into a whole. The whole consists on one level of their individualised narrative and, on another, of the encouragement towards a sense of belonging to a wider group of refugee children with distinct yet comparable experiences.

The programme Just Show Who You Are was developed subsequently and introduced into schools in reception centres where more newly arrived children were likely to lack the necessary verbal skills to engage in The World United. It uses non-verbal working methods such as playing, dancing, moving and creative expressions and is aimed at developing strengths in terms of a sense of safety, sense of identity and trust in self and others. Children learned to accept being touched by others, co-operation, skills in expression and the recollection of positive experiences. The target group was primary age children between seven and ten. The programme was developed by an art therapist and a play therapist but designed so that regular teachers could carry it out. The first session focuses on the issue of safety and uses a glove puppet of a turtle named Sang Baga. The facilitator acts out the story of the turtle who initially lives in a beautiful country but his home is swept away by storms. He has to swim to safety but in doing so finds himself in a new and strange land. To cope he hides and curls up in his shell and sings himself a song. The story continues in subsequent lessons where new themes are introduced through the allegorical tale of the turtle such as friendship and trust.

A further primary level programme was introduced in 2004 entitled Applause for Yourself and aimed at younger children aged between four and seven. This also used hand puppets but the central aim was to enhance the 'emotional competence' of the children. In particular, 'children can recognise their feelings and emotions, can mention them and can express their feelings'. The programme consists of nine weekly sessions involving the allegorical tale of a doll who takes the children on a 'discovery tour through a number of lands like the Land of Myself, You and Me, Glad, Angry, Sad and Afraid' (Pharos, 2007).

The same underlying principles inform the programmes for secondary level students. Central to these is the Refugee Lesson which was piloted in 1995, published in 1997, and has subsequently been used widely in schools with refugee children. A particular feature of this programme is that it was developed in a partnership between Pharos, a local comprehensive school and the local outpatient mental health services. While it was not designed for those adjudged to have severe behavioural problems or in need of psychiatric or psychothera-peutic help, it did focus on older children who seemed to need specific attention for social emotional problems. The Pharos manual suggests that those who would particularly benefit from it include students who show depressive behav-iour or other forms of mild psychological problems. The list also includes students who exhibit mild behavioural problems and a non-specified category of 'unaccompanied minors' (de Ruuk, 2002, p51). A teacher selects these stu-dents and, if they are willing to take part, they have a preliminary discussion of the programme with someone responsible for supervising it. The lessons are offered by a teacher or school counsellor and a professional from the field of mental health.

There are eight sessions conducted during school hours and lasting 50 min-utes each. The topics include: living in the Netherlands, where do I come from? who am I? important things and days, friendship and being in love, prospects for the future. As in the case of The World United, the sessions aim initially at building confidence before participants are invited to talk more openly about their experiences. There is a lessening of emotional intensity towards the end of the programme and refugee children are encouraged to end with positive atti-tudes towards oneself and others. In one session the focus is on the memories of the children and they are asked to make a drawing of a house in their country of origin. This forms the basis for a subsequent discussion. In another, the students are asked to bring in three objects that are important to them. De Ruuk records a session in which a girl brings in a shirt of a boyfriend who had died in Bosnia, provoking sympathy and support from the supervisor and members of the group.

Following the development of the Refugee Lesson, Pharos introduced a more general programme aimed at students from refugee and other backgrounds attending the international bridge classes. This programme, entitled Welcome to School, was not limited to a selected group but was made generally available for students up to 16 years old. It was considerably longer than the other school pro-grammes and extended to 21 weekly lessons covering broad themes such as 'getting to know each other, my country and the Netherlands, me and the people around me, and on the road to a future together'. Incorporated within these themes were weekly sessions on topics such as love, friendship, leisure time and health issues. The topics also included a session on 'exclusion' in which the young refugees explore experiences relating to racism and sex discrimination. In the example given in the manual, the topic explored is an incidence of sex dis-crimination in Afghanistan.

The two further programmes offered by Pharos are aimed directly at teachers. School as a Healer is a one-day course offered for those working with asylum seekers and refugees and examines salient risk and protective factors as well as related aspects of child development. The second part of the course is aimed at exploring the positive aspect of school in promoting the well-being of children and the roles teachers can play in enhancing this. The second teacher-focused programme is entitled Refugee Youth at School and is a manual for teacher training. Its aim is to enhance the skills of secondary school teachers so that they are as well equipped as possible to aid the reduction of socio-emotional problems in refugee children. The manual is used in a 'train the trainers' function with those experienced in the approach organising courses and training sessions. It is comparable to the 'Refugee Lesson' in that it has a strong focus on what may broadly be described as mental health aspects and supports training that is mostly done with mental health outpatient units. The training covers four topics: backgrounds of refugee youth, coping with losses, how to deal with traumatised children, and preventative activities in the classroom.

The Pharos school programmes are increasingly influential mechanisms for working with refugee children and have been the subject of some evaluation studies. These have produced varying results that, in turn, appear to be influenced by the methods used to conduct them. An initial quantitative study of the psychological impact of the Refugee Lesson, for example, showed no significant changes in the psychosocial adjustment of refugee children. However, a subsequent qualitative study showed that, from the perspectives of the refugee children themselves, the programme was meeting its objectives (de Ruuk, 2002). Pharos has reported on a study conducted between 2002 and 2004 which examined the outcomes of the programmes The World United and Just Show Who You Are, that appears to show that refugee children who participate in these programmes have both better well-being and improved cognitive abilities. In another study reported by Pharos, teachers did not note any significant behavioural improvement between a group who used the programme and one that did not. However, this contrasted with the results from students' own assessments of their well-being, which showed marked improvement on a well-being scale specifically on social functioning and a reduction in psychosomatic problems. These effects were not visible immediately after the end of programme but appeared one year later (Pharos, 2007; Ingleby and Watters, 2002).

It is difficult to draw definitive conclusions at this stage from these evaluations, as one would have to closely scrutinise the methods used and the data to form an objective judgement. Furthermore, as Ingleby has argued, in some cases programmes are felt to be beneficial by both the recipients and the facilitators while at the same time the results may not indicate clear improvements using standard psychological rating scales. In commenting on the results of two studies on the impact of two programmes of creative activities with refugee children in the Netherlands, Ingleby comments,

> our failure to detect psychological changes after activities which all concerned regard as extremely worthwhile and productive, may simply indicate

that we are looking for effects in the wrong places...children may have changed in ways that our scales cannot detect.

(Ingleby, 2005a, p179)

He argues that attention should be given to effects that are not normally taken into account such as the positive message that the programme gives to refugee children compared to 'the rejection they often experience at school, and the interminable trials and tribulations they suffer at the hands of the Dutch bureaucracy'. He adds that the programmes also have a beneficial effect on teachers that is not normally taken into account; 'several teachers in the project reported that giving the lessons had opened up new ways for them to relate to the children and had given them new perspectives on learning. That, surely, has to be regarded as a positive outcome' (ibid.).

More extensive evidence of the efficacy of school-based creative programmes is provided by Cecile Rousseau and her colleagues from Montreal Children's Hospital. They note that recorded benefits of therapy methods based on play and creative expression have included improved self-esteem, expression of emotions, problem solving and conflict resolution (Rousseau *et al.*, 2005, p180). There is research evidence of the effectiveness of this type of programme with at risk pre-school black children from deprived neighbourhoods and with children from families affected by alcohol or drug use. In extending the evaluation work to refugee and immigrant children, Rousseau and her colleagues note that challenges may be faced in working with this group in that they are culturally heterogeneous and highly varied in terms of their experiences in their homelands and in the post-migration environment. Secondly, the researchers were aware of the fact that the gap between school and the family was already wide and the programme could exacerbate this. Finally they noted that little was known in theory or practice about the activities that may work best.

The programmes described by Rousseau and her colleagues had been developed from pilot projects over a period of five years. The first of these was called The Trip in which children were asked to create a character of their choice who travels through a migration experience including the past, the trip itself, arrival in the host country and the future. A second project focused on two activities. In one children explored myths belonging to 'non-dominant' cultures (not necessarily their own) which represent, 'the tension and richness of the minority position'. In another they introduced myths and stories from their own communities which are more closely related to the children's identity. The activities were integrated into a final 12-week programme run by an art therapist and a psychologist with the teacher. The programme combined verbal and non-verbal means of expression such as painting or telling a story. Rousseau *et al.* describe the programme as having three aims:

to enable the children to create or recreate a meaningful and coherent world around their pre-migration and migration experience; to foster reciprocal respect of differences in identity and experience so as to promote bonding between children; and to bridge the gap between home and school.

(ibid., p181)

The evaluation centred on 138 children aged between 7 and 13 with a mean age of 9.8. Pre-test and post-test data was collected using three well established methods including an interactive version of DOMINIC, a children's self report (Scott *et al.*, 2006), a teachers report form developed by Achenbach, and the Piers-Harris Self-Concept scale used to measure the children's self-esteem (Rousseau *et al.*, 2005, p182). The results showed that the children who had undertaken the programme displayed lower mean scores for externalising (e.g. hyperactivity, conduct and oppositional disorders) and internalising (e.g. phobias, general anxiety, separation anxiety and depression) symptoms. They also had higher levels of feelings of popularity and satisfaction than children in control groups and higher levels of self-esteem, particularly for boys. The researchers conclude that 'the results of this evaluative study suggest that creative expression workshops have a positive effect on immigrant and refugee children's self esteem and may decrease their emotional and behavioural symptoms' (ibid., p183). Interestingly they noted that the positive effect on self-esteem was greater for boys and hypothesise that this may be due to 'the gap between boys' role models in their country of origin and the models provided by the host society' (ibid., p184). The impact of bridging the gap between the country of origin and the host society that is undertaken in the workshops may therefore be greater for boys.

Conclusion

The above examples are not, of course, the only examples of programmes for refugee children aimed at improving their psychological, social and emotional well-being. They are, however, particularly influential and informed by theoretical orientations common to many programmes. They have been carefully constructed and are often the product of many years of piloting different methods and careful reflection. From my own experience, those involved in them are strongly motivated by a desire to improve the mental health and well-being of refugee children. The programmes are broadly of the psychosocial 'type' identified by de Berry and reflect in their goals and methods many of the characteristics of resiliency among refugee children identified above, including cognitive and affective qualities listed, for example, by Apfel and Simon (2000). Despite the efforts of staff at Pharos and Rousseau and others, evaluation studies are still at a relatively early stage and there are concerns about the sustainability of beneficial effects some refugee children experience.

While it is important to recognise the potential benefits of the programmes, it is also essential to locate them within the wider discursive and institutional contexts in which they have been generated. In broad terms, the programmes offered by Pharos are integrationist in that they presuppose a one-way process of adaptation by the refugee children. The children are expected to integrate into a temporal sequencing of their experiences constructed by the teachers in which pre-migration, flight and post-migration experiences become 'whole'. The forming of an individualised narrative of their experiences is a central aspect of the programmes, as exemplified in the ME-books. The children are also taught to integrate with the group of other refugee children through exercises aimed at sharing experiences and building trust. The sessions provide structures that emphasise their commonalities, building on a template of the 'refugee experience' as consisting of pre-flight, flight, and post-flight experiences. Refugee children are here located within a social episteme in which they can be grouped together and offered programmes of collective treatment aimed at sharing and alleviating what service providers view as their common problems. Institutionally, they are situated between the domains of education and mental health care, with teachers developing a range of psychologically and psychotherapeutically oriented competences to deal with them.

It is notable how the terms 'social-emotional problems' and 'refugee children' are generated simultaneously and often uncritically in the policy and practice literature of special programmes. It is routinely assumed that refugee children are either suffering from social-emotional problems or are vulnerable to their development at a later stage, thus emphasising the importance of preventative strategies. The orientation here recalls Malkki's noting of what she describes as the thematic prominence of the 'psychological interpretation of displacement'. She cites Brik *et al.*'s observation that 'it is a generally accepted conclusion...that refugees constitute a high-risk group as far as mental health is concerned, due to the mere fact that they have been forced to emigrate'. Malkki adds that, 'We cannot assume psychological disorder or mental illness a priori, as an axiom, nor can we claim to know, from the mere fact of refugeeness, the actual sources of a person's suffering' (Malkki, 1995, p55). As noted above, this construction of refugee children as having actual or potential mental health problems is far from unique to the programmes discussed here and is common to a range of policy formulations in countries of reception. The programmes described, however, represent contexts in which this is operationalised in respect of refugee children in ways that are both tangible and influential.

Just as refugee children are homogenised as suffering from a range of analytically similar experiences and latent vulnerabilities, so they are decontextualised in that the programmes constitute them as a group outside of their families and cultural contexts. Indeed, one striking aspect of the Pharos programmes, as indeed of the descriptions of the problems of refugee children in other contexts, is the omission of reference to, or negative portrayal of, their parents. In the Pharos manual and publications there are numerous references to parents who are presented as, at best, inadequate, but often incompetent, negligent or even abusive. Owing to their own adverse experiences and the accumulation of stressors they have experienced, the parents are viewed as potentially moving from being a protective factor for the child to actually being a risk factor. A similar orientation is found in official literature on devitalisation. As noted, parents are described here as, in large proportion, 'insufficient, gravely mentally stressed or incapable of looking after their children, giving them hope or supporting them' (Hessle, 2005, p47). Thus families, far from being potential supports in the development of resilience, are seen as likely to have intensified the child's problems. This pathologising of parents is accompanied by a view of teachers as figures who can provide the children with positive adult role models.

Arguably, the bad parental practices recorded in some of the Pharos and devitalisation literature is genuinely reflective of aspects of the situation on the ground with parents and children in reception centres. However, this portrayal of parents is often insensitive to the highly demoralising and disempowering position they are placed in and the enormous challenges of raising children within environments over which they have little or no control. As a number of studies have shown, the asylum procedures adopted in industrialised countries are often themselves damaging to asylum seekers' mental health, contributing to states of anxiety and depression and exacerbating PTSD (Silove *et al.*, 2000). It would indeed be surprising if these did not result in fraught family units in which children were not brought up in an ideal way, both from the service providers *and* the parents' points of view.

A related area of concern is the routine superimposition of Westernised norms and values as evaluative mechanisms for assessing childcare practices on children who are from a variety of religious, ethnic and cultural backgrounds. The assertion that service providers should be sensitive to cultural factors is not tantamount to advocating a position of cultural relativism. Indeed, prominent critics of relativist positions recognise the importance of respect for individual and group autonomy. As Ignatieff has argued, advocates of human rights must support and enhance individual agency and, at a collective level, 'must respect the rights of those groups to define the type of collective life they wish to lead, provided that this life meets the minimalist standards requisite to the enjoyment of human rights at all' (Ignatieff, 2001, p18). Within these parameters, human rights practice must go beyond, 'the vague requirement to display cultural sensitivity' and is 'obliged to seek consent for its norms and to abstain from interference when consent is not freely given (ibid.). While consent is sought for participation in the programmes described above, the role of parents appears to have minimal influence in the formulation of programmes, and in relation to wider participation and evaluation. Moreover, the programmes here are targeted at individual children who are incorporated into groups of 'refugee children' in ways that reflect the categories and presuppositions of service providers. They are not targeted at seeking to enhance the functioning of groupings defined by the refugees themselves and do not appear to engage with cultural processes that are collectively meaningful to the refugees.

An underlying assumption is that children have been subject to debilitating ruptures in their lives and the programmes will help to make them whole again by linking together the strands of past, present and future and through becoming part of an emotionally supportive group of refugee children. It is interesting that the salient grouping is that of refugee children rather than what may be more natural groups based on family, kinship or ethnicity. The children are taught through the programmes to view themselves as part of an international group, the cohesiveness of which is not generated though traditional moral or affective ties, but through a view that this constructed group has similar problems and vulnerabilities. The children may thus be viewed as undergoing two core displacements, an original one in which they have left their homes and countries of origin, and a second one in which they gradually disengage from the family and cultural groupings they are familiar with, to be re-embedded into a new identity and collectivity conforming to the structures and categories of the host society.

There is insufficient evidence available at present to assess the longer-term impact of the programmes and, as Ingleby has observed, one should be cautious in formulating evaluative criteria (Ingleby, 2005a). It may be, for example, that as a consequence of the programme the children feel more integrated into Dutch society. Simultaneously, they may also feel more distant from their parents and the culture and customs they grew up with. As Rousseau has cautioned, the programme devised by host country therapists and educators 'could easily become just one more disparate element in the children's two separate worlds' (Rousseau *et al.*, 2005, p181). If evaluation criteria reflects only the concerns of institutions in the host society, it may well provide evidence of 'success' that does not reflect the concerns of the refugee children themselves or of their families.

The issue of the extent of engagement with parents is a complex one that arguably further supports the argument for mainstreaming refugee children in host society schools. The disjunction between educational services and parents appears to be greatest when the latter are placed in residential centres and their children in special schools or classes that are isolated from the mainstream. In the examples cited above from the UK and Belgium, schools have made particular efforts to engage with parents and this aspect appears as a cornerstone of good practice. Where the opportunity has presented itself, the parents of refugee children have shown that they can be active and engaged in their child's educational progress. The Canadian studies referred to above suggest examples of programmes that do engage with parents both in establishing the programme and in its evaluation. A potentially fruitful area of future research would be a comparative study of programmes with and without parental involvement.

The examples discussed here have much in common with a variety of special programmes for refugee children and suggest the following characteristics:

- an overriding emphasis on psycho-social or psycho-emotional problems
- an emphasis on the development of individualising narratives linking past, present and future
- an emphasis on encouraging bonds of empathy and affinity with a wider community of refugee children
- an emphasis on one-way integration and adaptation.

Within these programmes the refugee child is viewed as living in a shattered world that needs to be made whole. The making whole can be seen as having both a vertical and a horizontal dimension. The vertical dimension relates to temporal aspects of the refugee child's experiences and the construction of a linear chronology linked to a concept of personal integration. The horizontal dimension links the refugee child to the wider community of refugee children with whom he or she is encouraged to integrate through recognition of a commonality of experience. Besides the more obviously psychological influences on the programmes, their orientation has arguably an implicit theological underpinning. While we cannot pursue the matter in any depth here, it is notable that concepts of personal integration linking past, present and future are close to

Christian notions of salvation. As noted by one eminent theologian, 'human beings have always been in a quest for salvation, of making whole what is broken in existence' (Fiddes, 1989). Fiddes notes that 'Salvation is an idea that has the widest scope, including the healing of individuals and social groups'. Similarly, the social integration encouraged through the programmes is arguably close to traditional concepts of 'atonement' or 'making as one'. Whether or not the programmes are implicitly or explicitly influenced by these concepts is a matter of conjecture. However, it is important to recognise that the theories and processes involved in them do not themselves stand outside of historical and cultural influences.

Good practice in services for refugee children

The preceding chapters have provided an overview of some of the salient issues relating to the reception, education and social care of refugee children. On the basis of the examination of host countries' responses, it is possible to provide an outline of principles of good practice. These will be identified and explored in the context of an examination of macro, meso and micro aspects. Specifically, six elements of good practice are identified here; access and entitlement, participation, holistic practice, interagency collaboration, cultural sensitivity and reflexivity, and evaluation. These are examined in turn to highlight salient issues relating to research and practice. The chapter will conclude with consideration of the potential for transferring good practice from one reception country to another.

The question of good practice

There have been numerous reports and policy guidelines on the subject of promoting good practice for refugees and some that have emphasised practice in relation to refugee children. The notion of good practice is underpinned by an evaluative judgement that not only is the practice identified as 'good', but often that it represents an example that should be adopted elsewhere. Policy recommendations are often interspersed with examples of good practice. In national documents these are usually drawn from examples from around a particular country, while international documents draw examples from various countries. To take an example discussed earlier, the report of the Audit Commission in the UK into the implications of the dispersal of asylum seekers contained numerous 'case studies' of good practice in services for asylum seekers from regions that formed a basis for the formulation of wider policy recommendations (Audit Commission, 2000). A 2006 report by the Austrian and European Red Cross and supported by the European Commission into the reception and health care of refugees lists some 40 examples of 'good practice' from across the European Union (Red Cross, 2006). The European Council on Refugees and Exiles has produced a series of good practice guides relating to aspects of refugee integration in Europe, covering items such as health, education, housing, community and culture (www.ecre.org).

While much of this endeavour produces a useful exchange of information on developments in different countries and regions, it tells us little about the contexts in which projects have been developed, how they are located within the health and social care systems of particular countries, their sustainability and how they are viewed by those who use them. I have argued elsewhere that the context in which services are developed is of vital importance in determining their quality and sustainability. Furthermore, services for minority ethnic groups were often developed in the context of short-term projects that had a marginal status in relation to mainstream provision (Watters, 1996a). Thus, while very good services may be delivered through a project, the wider institutional position of the project could militate against its medium and long-term impact. Further research indicates that these problems are likely to be present in many of the services targeted at refugees (Watters *et al.*, 2003). The position of these services arguably reflects and reproduces the wider position of the client groups they seek to serve with marginal groups receiving services that are themselves marginal.

Recognition of the interrelationship between the institutional context of a service and its capacity to deliver services to marginalised groups has methodological and analytical implications. For one, it suggests that linkages should be explored between the level at which services are delivered and a macro level at which they are established and funded. I have referred elsewhere to this as an 'institutional level' (Watters, 2001a). An intermediate level, referred to elsewhere as the 'service level', relates to an examination of how the service operates in relation to other organisations within its locality and sphere of activity. The proposal that services for refugee children should be examined through macro, meso and micro levels is not to imply that these levels are in any way separate. The purpose is rather the reverse; to provide an analytic framework for exploring how they are interrelated. The principles behind this framework are of central importance in the study of good practice.

To take one hypothetical but not atypical example, a mental health project for refugees may produce evidence of good clinical outcomes. The service has been created through a funding partnership involving national and regional government and an NGO. The funding itself is based on generalised views of the primary needs of asylum seekers and refugees and of the professional bodies and specialisms best equipped to meet those needs. By placing an emphasis on supporting victims of torture and refugee children, it was hoped to minimise potential government and public hostility and maximise the chances of support. The service was not developed on the basis of an assessment of the overall needs of the potential client group or on any forms of consultation. The parameters of the evaluation were constructed around measurable clinical outcomes and these in turn provided ongoing justification for the continuation of the project. The project was routinely cited as an example of good practice and one that was influential in the establishment of similar projects elsewhere. This not atypical example demonstrates the circularity of logic noted by Castles and referred to in Chapter 1. Here policy driven and narrowly focused empirical research 'accepts the problem definitions built into its terms of reference, and does not look for more fundamental causes, nor for more challenging solutions' (Castles, 2003, p26).

A multi-level approach towards identifying good practice provides an opportunity to examine it from broader perspectives and assess performance on the basis of wider criteria. An emphasis solely on clinical outcomes tells us little about how the provision of the service matches the needs of victims of torture and refugee children within its catchment area. Broader questions that could be included within a consideration of good practice are:

- How accessible is the intervention?
- How are the needs or wishes of users reflected in the intervention?
- To what extent have users influenced, directly or indirectly, the form of the activity?
- How much attention, and what kind, is paid to possible effects of cultural differences?
- Is the intervention original?
- Are attempts made to evaluate the success of the intervention?

(Watters *et al.*, 2003, p10)

To these could be added further questions relating to the macro and meso levels, for example:

- To what extent is the service based on existing knowledge regarding the needs of the client group it seeks to serve?
- How is the service funded and what limitations does this place on the delivery of services?
- How does the service interrelate with other agencies involved in providing services to the client group?

While these questions may appear both self-evident and important, they are rarely considered in formulating criteria for assessing good practice. Where wider macro and structural aspects are taken into consideration this is usually in the context of descriptive accounts of projects rather than as aspects of its evaluation. So, for example, recent surveys of good practice in the refugee field undertaken by the European Council for Refugees and Exiles (ECRE) and by the Red Cross provide information on funding and institutional partnerships supporting initiatives (Red Cross, 2006). However, the emphasis in determining good practice often rests simply on accounts given by the organisations themselves with these items providing background information. The ECRE may list aspects such as a lack of sustainable funding as a negative feature of a project, but this is not done in any systematic or comprehensive way. These observations are not intended as criticisms of what are well intentioned and useful endeavours, but are rather aimed at pointing to more generic problems in much of the policy-oriented literature on good practice.

In undertaking a major international study into the mental health and social care of refugees a wide range of sources and criteria for good practice were investigated.

These included national standards for health and social care provision, the findings of working groups convened by NGOs, specially commissioned reports into services for refugees and evidence of the views of service users themselves (Watters *et al.*, 2003). Drawing on this material and on the recommendations of further reports and guidelines on refugee children, the following matrix of good practice is proposed. Essentially its elements are as follows:

- access and entitlement
- participation
- holistic practice
- interagency collaboration
- cultural sensitivity and reflexivity
- evaluation.

Each of these elements of good practice are examined in turn, drawing out salient issues for research and service development.

Access and entitlement

This aspect concerns the way in which services reach refugee children and refugee children reach services. As noted, questions of access are complex and should be distinguished analytically from questions of entitlement. These two elements are routinely conflated in policy statements and country descriptions of the situation of asylum seekers and refugees. Put crudely, entitlement relates to questions at a macro level concerning laws and policies, while access relates to actual practice on the ground. The question as to whether refugee children have entitlement to a particular service, for example, education or health care, can be answered by reference to bodies of official literature. The question of access, on the other hand, requires examination into the implementation of laws and policies at what Lipsky would describe as 'street level' (1980). In some countries, for example the UK, there is relatively wide entitlement to services for asylum seekers and refugees. However, in practice gaining access may be problematic as semi-independent actors such as GPs or school headmasters may be constrained in providing primary health care or school admission for a variety of reasons. Access is also limited by the profile of services in particular areas. The introduction, for example, of a specialist mental health team to work with refugees may mean that many refugees have access to this particular service. The cutting of funding to the team may result in this access being denied. As such, questions regarding the extent to which refugee children can gain access to services goes beyond legal entitlement to meso-level questions regarding the variety of appropriate agencies within particular localities and patterns of referral between them. This in turn is linked to questions of the social construction of refugees' problems and needs, as this determines the provision of particular types of services. There may be, for example, potentially very good access to services for refugees suffering from PTSD in Stockholm and Montreal, but poor access to welfare advice and accommodation.

The questions of access and entitlement are therefore fundamental to good practice. Put simply, if a service is adjudged to offer good practice to refugee children it should be based on fundamental entitlement, but offer at 'street level' access for children. Access in this sense may be characterised as having both an 'active' and a 'protective' aspect. Its active component relates to questions of outreach and the ready availability of information on the service in appropriate places. An example of an active approach to access in this sense is provided by the Platform for Reception of Unaccompanied Minors in Paris. The platform represents a co-ordinated programme of activity directed at unaccompanied minors by five NGOs including accommodation, legal advice, administrative support for access to health care, French language courses, legal representation and financial aid. The five NGOs involved have differing levels of experience and resources for meeting the needs of minors in these areas. The combination of their efforts represents a 'client-led' approach – it is the needs of the clients that are determining the configuration of services. Two of the NGOs on the platform, Arc 75 and Hors la Rue have expertise in working with minors living on the streets and offering them practical support. Their modus operandi includes trying first to set up a relation of trust with the minor, making an evaluation of his or her situation, providing accommodation in accordance with the places available, supplying food, legal and medical support (Red Cross, 2006, p31).

What may be described as a more 'protective' approach relates to not erecting barriers towards refugee children's access to services. This may mean countering measures designed to introduce newly imposed restrictions. The emphasis here is on seeking to ensure that levels of access are maintained, often in political environments in which new constraints are being introduced. Again, the relationship with entitlement is important to note here as oppositional measures towards restrictions in entitlement require challenges to the introduction of new laws and policies. A protective role suggests the work of activists and lobbyists, while the maintenance of access implies grassroots advocacy.

Participation

The importance of participation is highlighted in the Convention on the Rights of the Child (CRC) where no less than four articles outline children's rights to participate. According to Article 12, 'States Parties shall assure to the child who is capable of forming his or her own views the right to express those views freely in all matters affecting the child, the views of the child being given due weight in accordance with the age and maturity of the child'. The article continues,

> For this purpose, the child shall in particular be provided the opportunity to be heard in any judicial and administrative proceedings affecting the child, either directly, or through a representative or an appropriate body, in a manner consistent with the procedural rules of national law.
>
> (UN, 1989)

In *The State of the World's Children* published by UNICEF in 2003, it is argued that the purpose behind the CRC articles on participation is 'to optimise opportunities for meaningful participation' (cited by Ansell, 2005, p236). Ansell has noted that the idea of children's participation now receives international support with the UN defining youth participation as having four components: economic, social, political and cultural participation. She argues that 'not only do children have the interest and capacity to participate in decision making, their involvement brings wide-ranging benefits' (ibid., p235). These include improved decision making in matters affecting children that lay strong foundations for the development of active citizenship in later life. Literature on the mental health of refugees suggests further that the participation of refugees in programmes may also have good mental health outcomes and should be encouraged.

Roger Hart's 'ladder of participation' provides an oft-cited model for the evaluation of levels of participation. It moves from three lower rungs that are not considered to be beneficial, namely manipulation, decoration and tokenism, to more desirable higher rungs. The latter, in ascending order, are 'assigned but informed, consulted and informed, adult-initiated, shared decisions with children, child-initiated', and finally 'child-initiated, shared decisions with adults' (Hart, 1992). It has been noted that one benefit of the model is that 'it demonstrates how some processes that are claimed as participatory involve minimal or no change in power relations' (Laws *et al.*, 2003, p61). However, Laws and her colleagues have argued that the hierarchical image does not address the complexities of programmes: 'It tends to suggest that whatever the situation, greater participation is desirable, with the final goal being autonomous organising by the group in question' (ibid.). They suggest a more nuanced approach that recognises different levels of participation as appropriate at different stages of a project (ibid., p62).

While recognising the merits of this criticism, Hart's ladder does have the further benefit of drawing a distinction between participation in a predefined programme and having a role in shaping the programme itself. To take the example of the Pharos programmes described in Chapter 6, they are designed and initiated by psychologists and teachers, and children are presented with a clearly structured programme of activity, with topics that are covered and rituals that begin and end the sessions. These are a 'given' within which children are invited to participate. In this context they participate in a limited sense in, for example, choosing objects that reflect their experiences and telling their own stories. Approaching Hart's level of 'adult-initiated, shared decisions with children', implies that children have a say in the topics to be covered in a programme and perhaps also in its overall structure.

However, the construction of a dichotomised model consisting only of interfaces between adults and children does not reveal the stresses and complexities arising from questions of participation. It is more helpful here to consider a triangular relationship involving children, parents and service providers. In some initiatives, for example, the schools programmes referred to above in the UK, Canada and Belgium, do have strong links to parents, who are consulted over aspects of their children's schooling. Some of the measures introduced were concerned with strengthening the position of parents by acquainting them with the books and technology their children would be using and offering them access to learning resources in schools. Through these measures, refugee children's parents were empowered to support their children at school, and potential divisions between family and school were minimised. Parental participation is not, of course, equivalent to the participation of children themselves but is, I would argue, in most cases of benefit to children. One could envisage situations in which parents or services used opportunities for participation to undermine children, but these are likely to be exceptions.

Jo de Berry and her colleagues in their study of children's lives in Kabul offer a radical perspective on children's participation. Here children were seen not 'as passive recipients of support but as active individuals who play an important role in their own development, relationships and protection' (de Berry *et al.*, 2003, p2). The researchers invoke the emphasis noted above in the Convention on the Rights of the Child on participation and the consequent emphasis placed on this aspect by UNICEF and Save the Children. Rather than entering Kabul with predefined notions of what the children's problems were and how they would help them, de Berry *et al.* oriented their study towards gaining an understanding of the values and practices that the children used to sustain their own lives, and to offer support in ways the children themselves indicated would be helpful. In research terms, their approach could be described as 'emic' rather than 'etic' in that the emphasis was on understanding and employing the categories participants used to make sense of their lives, rather than those imposed through an external scientific discourse. Following Giddens, another way to describe the approach is that it employed a 'single' rather than a 'double' hermeneutic in that the ordinary language of the participants was itself the object of study and the tool for analysis and action rather than a secondary rendition, say, into discourses associated with psychology or social work (Giddens, 1984).

The participatory methods employed in the programme included eliciting the children's own concepts relating to aspects of life such as well-being and happiness. 'Tariba', for example, emerged as a particularly important concept for the children. It referred to 'children's manners and the quality of their relationships with others'. Those with good tariba were described as 'polite, obedient, respectful, sociable and peaceful' while those with bad tariba were 'rude, antisocial and argumentative' (de Berry *et al.*, 2003). The researchers explored key values and concepts with children and also in groups of fathers and mothers. They found that there was often overlap between the perspectives of children and their families, with qualities such as tariba and delair (courage) being seen as highly desirable by all groups. Parents and children had holistic views of what constituted well-being, incorporating physical, social, emotional and religious qualities. Feelings were seen as not only related to emotional or mental health but were experienced in and through the body, 'a child who has good and positive feelings will be healthy, while a child who has negative feelings will be simultaneously sick and weak'. The authors conclude that, 'people in Kabul understand that negative feelings are somatised – they result in physical conditions' (de Berry *et al.*, 2003, p11). It is notable that this general view of the interrelationship between mind, emotions and the body is confirmed in some contemporary areas of medical research in, for example, the field of psychoneuroimmunology (e.g. Kiecolt *et al.*, 1998). They also correspond to many contemporary approaches to therapy in the industrialised world represented as 'holistic', for example combined approaches incorporating physical, emotional and social work. The authors referred to a 'remarkable consistency' in these views expressed by groups in different parts of Kabul.

One aspect of life that was considered highly important by both parents and children was the undertaking of household tasks. These were seen as vital in the development of skills for later life and were often a source of pride rather than resentment among children. Indeed, the successful undertaking of these tasks featured in the 'happy day' stories researchers elicited from the children.

> Children said that when these roles go well – when they are easily able to collect water, or when a chicken in their care has chicks – they feel especially happy. Regarding the common task of collecting water, children were happy to undertake it because it was helpful to their family but were also worried about the dangers that may arise from mines, traffic and the lack of infrastructure resulting from prolonged armed conflict and bombings.
>
> (de Berry *et al.*, 2003, p13)

De Berry and her colleagues' descriptions of the work undertaken by children and the children's relation to it, recalls Scheper-Hughes and Sargent's discussion of child labour in other international contexts. Citing evidence from fieldwork in Zimbabwe and New Mexico, the authors point to examples of the sense of usefulness and respect children can gain from supporting their families through their labour. As noted in Chapter 2, they challenge prevailing Western notions of child labour as being necessarily a bad thing and point to the paradoxical attitudes found in many affluent societies where discourses of child centredness are combined with prevailing views of children as a burden and economic liability. They suggest that a conceptually useful way forward is to differentiate 'child *work* within the context of families and home communities from child *labour* within the context of industrial and global capitalism' (Scheper-Hughes and Sargent, 1998, p12, emphasis in original).

While the successful undertaking of work for the family was viewed by children as contributing to their happiness, this was one aspect of a broader view of the factors that contribute to well-being. De Berry and colleagues summarise the range of factors that contribute to well-being as; 'gained through historical events which change things for the better, a conducive environment enabling them to fulfil roles and responsibilities; opportunities for self development and, most important of all, relationships with other people, especially their families' (2003, p14). One aspect of these relationships is defined as 'wasta', a concept that refers to a situation in which family members are in good jobs and with good connections and appears not dissimilar to notions of social capital. Indeed the concept is highly significant in Arab societies with Cunningham and Sarayrah asserting that 'Understanding wasta is key to understanding decisions in the Middle East, for wasta pervades the culture of all Arab countries and is a force in every significant decision…Wasta is a way of life' (Cunningham and Sarayrah, 1993, p3). In academic literature in the Middle East the concept is routinely referred in terms of the role of networks in achieving economic and social advantages such as gaining access to particular types of employment (see for example, Denoeux, 2005).

The participatory methods employed by de Berry and colleagues reveal concepts of well-being inextricably linked to ties with extended family members and neighbours. In the case of the Afghan children they researched, loss and separation from family members was construed as the biggest threat children could face, and highly damaging to well-being. By undertaking in-depth research with the children, the researchers constructed a map of salient personal, social and environmental issues that were of concern and subsequently used these as a basis for developing programmes of action to address perceived problems. These drew on community members including parents, children and local religious leaders and identified measures to improve road safety, neighbourhood campaigns to reduce physical threats like open wells and rubbish dumps and child-focused landmine education. Measures also included strengthening health professionals' capacities to 'recognise and treat psychosocial needs by encouraging social or religious coping mechanisms and not prescribing drugs – especially for children' (de Berry *et al.*, 2003, p62).

Following the phase of research that resulted in the production of the *Children of Kabul* report, the researchers adopted a subsequent 'Child-to-Child' programme. This approach has been described as one that 'encourages children to find out more about the issues that concern them and to bring about action that will make the situation better'. The approach is as follows:

> Children work in groups in a Child-to-Child programme and, together, the group goes through six steps. In the first step, the groups think about the topic they are concerned about. In step two, children go out and find out more information about the problem. In step three, they think about ways to present the information they have about their concern. In step four, children present this information to their community using a variety of methods such as role plays or maps or posters. Finally, in step five, children take action on the problem, and in step six the children evaluate what impact their action has had.
>
> (de Berry, 2003, p72)

The approach has been adopted since the 1970s and at the time of writing has been introduced in over 80 countries with UNESCO and UNICEF among others. It has been the subject of a number of evaluations, including a comprehensive study undertaken between 1986 and 1990. This included qualitative and quantitative data collection in seven localities. According to an extensive review of the approach undertaken by Pridmore and Stephens, 'The evaluation concluded that Child-to-Child was an effective way to bring health messages to children, particularly in schools, and that it was sustainable because it was continuing in all the settlings evaluated after evaluation funding had ceased' (Pridmore and Stephens, 2000, p13). On the basis of this evaluation, Pridmore and Stephens identified a series of factors necessary for its successful implementation. These included staff participation at all levels and stages of decision making, an agreed definition of what a Child-to-Child approach means, acknowledgement of the gap between what teachers had been doing and what they were required to do, flexibility in the application of the approach, administrative support, ongoing evaluation and feedback during the process and engagement with topics that were relevant to children's situations. It has been, in particular, employed in the health care field and views children as having the potential to be actively involved in promoting the health of themselves and their peers (ibid.).

The *Children of Kabul* study represents one example of the ways in which a broad participatory approach has been successfully adopted within a major contemporary refugee-producing country, and one from which a high proportion of refugee children originate. The methods employed in the study indicate some of the fruitful ways in which a participatory and consultative process can be employed with children. In practice, there are a number of initiatives that employ a participatory approach as described here. Giorgia Dona has described various contexts in which children have been engaged in participatory research. These have included a study by MacMullin and Loughry of the worries of Palestinian children living in Gaza, in which the children themselves were involved in the development of research instruments. They were asked to

> list and rank the things that worried them most, which constituted the basis for the development of a questionnaire that was distributed to 247 children aged 11 to 16, and whose findings were discussed in focus group meetings with the children themselves.
>
> (Dona, 2006, p23)

It is notable that in the study what Dona describes as 'different and unexpected' concerns became apparent including corruption, dirty streets, the future, death of Iraqi children and car accidents. Some of these reflect concerns expressed in Kabul and demonstrate the ways in which children are engaged both with the 'here and now' of their lives and broader issues that provoke their empathy. The formulation of problems challenges the homogenising and rather one-dimensional representation of refugee children as preoccupied solely with the effects of war and displacement and their traumatic effects.

In a further study, Dona examined the impact of fostering on Rwandan children who had become internally displaced or refugees as a result of the 1994 genocide. Despite efforts by the government and international organisations to reunite children with their families, tens of thousands remained separated,

> children too young to remember who they were or where they came from at the time of separation, and those for whom tracing had been unsuccessful, remained in centres or in the care of unrelated individuals both in Rwanda and abroad.
>
> (Dona, 2006, p25)

The latter was referred to as 'spontaneous' or informal fostering as contrasted with a subsequent programme in which agencies arranged 'formal' fostering. UNICEF and Save the Children commissioned the study to explore children's experiences of fostering. The approach described by Dona was widely participative in that it involved an advisory group consisting of children who influenced aspects of the methodology and scope of the study, including the choosing of representatives from among the children who would represent their views. The research included individual interviews and group work which extended to involving the children in aspects of the interpretation of findings. Dona gives the following example:

> we had encountered cases of unaccompanied children who had not been told they had been fostered (some of them had found out indirectly but pretended they did not know, while others believed themselves to be natural children). We had also found out that some foster parents, given the negative connotation that 'orphan' carries in post-genocide Rwanda, considered the fact that the child did not know a sign of success. It's difficult to strike a balance between the Convention (on the Rights of the Child) right to an identity, the implications of the label 'orphan' and the parents concerns about discrimination.
>
> (Ibid., p27)

Following consultation with the children it was concluded that children should know they had been fostered because it would avoid the child being told by an outsider and avoid problems concerning inheritance following the death of the parents. They advised that the children should be told sensitively, possibly by the parents themselves. The researchers also consulted the children about the structure of the report from the study and they suggested more emphasis should be placed on the future of the fostered children. Dona describes a process that was both enlightening and fulfilling for the researchers and for the children themselves, resulting in a sensitive and insightful piece of work.

While the concerns may be different to those of refugee children in industrialised countries, the potential benefit of adopting a participatory approach remains significant. One further example relates to the widespread view among service providers that they have not had enough training to meet clients' cultural needs (Watters, 2002b). These views have been expressed in the contexts of evaluative studies of services that offer little ongoing consultation with refugees themselves. One potential pitfall of training is that it can have the effect of reinforcing cultural stereotypes and homogenising refugee populations. Furthermore, training drawing on the expertise of one discipline can skew the view of refugee children to focus for example on clinical problems. This is not to suggest that all training does this, but that it is an area requiring careful consideration by those sponsoring programmes. A key consideration here is the utilisation of refugees and refugee children themselves as experts in their own culture and needs, rather than the assumption of the need for external expertise. This type of participation could be offered in the context of informal information sharing groups and would have the additional value of making the refugees themselves feel valued and trusted.

Holistic practice

A further aspect of good practice proposed here is the adoption of a holistic approach. Such an approach has been alluded to at various points in this book and it has been the aspiration of a number of policies and programmes targeting refugee children. Put simply, holistic practice may be defined as an approach that integrates aspects of social, emotional and psychological care and relates closely to the concept of a psychosocial approach as advocated, for example, by de Berry and her colleagues (de Berry *et al.*, 2003). More generally, holistic practice can be found in many areas of social care. Gunaratnam has noted, for example, its presence in hospice care where it is seen as 'subverting the traditional biomedical focus on social care needs through models of holistic care that aim to take account of the physical, emotional, spiritual and social needs of service users' (Gunaratnam, 2004, p117). Its numerous applications are supported by rapidly expanding bodies of research into the interrelationship between emotional, social and psychological conditions. Goldberg and Huxley, for example, have combined evidence of these interrelationships into what they have defined as a bio-social model in mental health care, while Brown and Harris established in the 1970s the relationships between social factors and depression (Goldberg and Huxley, 1994; Brown and Harris, 1978). As noted, advances in the field of psychoneuroimmunology have identified links between emotional and cognitive factors and the onset of physical illnesses (Lyon, 1993).

Many programmes targeting refugees in general and refugee children in particular explicitly endorse a holistic approach. However, what this actually means in practice can vary in emphasis from programme to programme and place to place. In broad terms, the approach is referred to in instances in which services include a broad assessment of refugee clients' needs including legal, social, health care and accommodation. This is the sense, for example, in which the AMBER project in Austria uses the term when referring to its 'holistic social counselling'. However, the social and holistic aspect is here quite circumscribed and the project is staffed by medical personnel and volunteers and is aimed at facilitating access to medical services and prevention for those who are excluded from the mainstream system (Red Cross, 2006, p11).

The term is also used, for example, in relation to Apanemi, a woman's information and support centre in Cyprus which runs a particular programme for refugees and asylum seekers. The aim of this service is described as enabling asylum seekers and refugees 'to be informed and facilitated in accessing their legal and human rights. The approach is holistic and participatory with special emphasis on gender-related violence and support for vulnerable groups' (Red Cross, 2006, p22). Here much of the work appears to be directed at enhancing the capacity of existing services, through co-ordination and training so that a comprehensive programme of care and support could be provided. This includes shelter from domestic violence, clothing and food, housing, GP visits and social and psychological counselling. The range of activity here is vast, with holistic care referring to the meeting of a comprehensive spectrum of material and psychosocial needs.

Indeed, the scope of projects is often partly or wholly determined by the circumscribed nature of government provision. It is notable that in some countries the provision of very basic supports to asylum seekers, for example accommodation and health care, is the province of NGOs operating special projects. In Denmark, the government refused to sign the EC directive on asylum reception and contracts the Red Cross to provide the ongoing operation of asylum centres. This includes the provision of housing, allowances, schools, kindergartens, job training, adult education, health care and social assistance. In Greece, the Hellenic Red Cross also provides or supervises a similarly wide range of activities at asylum reception centres. There is also a major role for NGOs in the provision of basic facilities, often in the context of contracts with the government in a range of asylum reception countries including the UK, the US and Australia. In this broader political context, the provision of holistic care may be a consequence of the restrictive parameters of care directly provided by governments. Here questions of the evaluation of good practice relate to the manner in which holistic care is provided, rather than being based on an assumption that the provision of a holistic approach in this sense is necessarily in itself a positive feature of services.

More specifically, the development of a holistic approach implies a service that is receptive to the needs of clients and is flexible in meeting those needs. However, the question of receptivity to needs is a complex one and, as Baldwin has argued, includes needs that are defined by experts and those defined by the clients themselves (Baldwin, 1998, p4). Here emphasis on holistic practice is linked to an emphasis on participation as explored above and engagement with refugee children in seeking to identify their needs. It does not imply a dogmatic approach in which a holistic programme is formulated based on an a priori view of what refugee children 'need' and which is then delivered to them come what may. Rather, it implies a situation in which a range of resources is potentially available and these are offered depending on the expressed needs of the child. It also implies that the child is informed as well as possible about the range of options he or she may have open to her. This approach is appropriately informed by a Maslowian conception of a hierarchy of needs consisting of physiological, safety, love, esteem and self-actualisation needs. This framework can be helpful in checking an impulse to focus initially on mental health programmes while refugee children may have more fundamental needs for housing and security. Again the emphasis here is on receptivity and flexible service provision and a hierarchical model may have to be adapted in the light of the expressed needs of children.

Interagency collaboration

The exhortation for agencies to work together and form 'partnerships' to address potentially intractable social problems such as drug addiction and homelessness is commonplace in the language of policy formation and practice. To take one of the potentially innumerable examples, the Social Inclusion Board of South Australia addressed the question of 'good practice in multi-agency linkages' in a governmental report on addressing the problems of homelessness (Social Inclusion

Board, 2003). The concepts of multi-agency linkages and interagency collaboration are also ubiquitous in the refugee field with interagency work seen as critical to the achievement of core national and international objectives. UNHCR, for example, routinely invokes the need for interagency collaboration in achieving durable solutions for refugees (UNHCR, 2006b). In terms of forming a measure for good practice, interagency collaboration implies more than the fact that an agency has links with others but that it actively works together with them in the pursuit of common goals.

It is helpful to note at least three ways in which this collaboration may manifest. One, which may be described as *formative* interagency collaboration, is where a programme is initiated through interagency collaboration involving, for example, a group of stakeholders who act as a management or steering group for the development of a project. Another, which may be described as *reactive*, is where collaborative interagency work is developed owing to the nature of the demands on a service exceeding its capacities. A further example may be described as *informal* where links are less formal and collaboration operates at a 'street level' where agencies combine to meet the needs of refugee clients. As such, collaboration can be construed as operating on macro or meso levels with the first example relating more clearly to macro-level practices and the second two to the meso level.

An example of the application of a formative approach is the Safe Case Transfer programme which, as noted above, involved the collaboration of a number of agencies in a project involving the transfer of unaccompanied asylum-seeking children from the south east of England to Manchester. The initiation of the programme was a consequence of joint work between local authority consortia in the Manchester area, Kent County Council in the south east and expertise provided by key NGOs and the Home Office. In practice, at various stages the initiative combined types of interagency collaboration identified above. An interagency steering group oversaw the management and evaluation of the project, while a range of formal and informal arrangements were made on the ground to ensure the refugee children had access to a full range of services such as legal support, health care, education, housing and welfare benefits.

Interagency collaboration at what may be described as 'street level' typically involves a case worker whose role includes the assessment of the refugee's needs and eliciting the support of a range of agencies with resources that can address a variety of material, health and social care aspects. An example can be drawn here from the Bi-cultural Team based at the Refugee Council in London (Watters *et al.*, 2003). Following an initial assessment of needs undertaken at the organisation's reception, those who appear to have mental health problems are referred to the team who undertake a more comprehensive assessment. On the basis of this, a range of approaches may be adopted. The team member may offer a series of counselling sessions combined with help with practical matters as well as providing a resource for ongoing contact. If the client appears to need help from other agencies there are a range of options for referral. Those who appear to have been victims of torture are referred to the Medical Foundation for the Care of Victims of Torture, who offer an in-depth assessment and also a range of therapeutic options. Often clients have a complex range of needs met by engaging with a variety of agencies involving, for example, making links with GPs, accommodation providers, legal support and possibly also schools and colleges. The model here recalls aspects of the integrated approach described by Silove and his colleagues at the University of New South Wales, as it incorporates both an aspect of direct psychosocial care provision as well as a capacity to offer outreach to a range of agencies (Silove *et al.*, 1999).

As noted above, while the principle of interagency collaboration remains central to a number of initiatives relating to refugee children, the content and context of the collaboration can be very different depending on wider political, legal and economic factors. Those working in the field are constantly navigating a nebulous interface between legal and welfare agencies in which there is an absence of clear policies on how to proceed. In the examples noted earlier in this book of children found in lorries at the port of Zeebrugge in Belgium, police had relatively weak links with many key agencies making help with health care and accommodation hard to achieve. A child protection officer could be contacted but in many instances this just resulted in children being released without any child protection measures being taken. The examples from a range of countries point to the importance of those who are directly at the interface with refugee children – at what we have defined as the micro level – having access to a range of reliable resources.

Cultural sensitivity and reflexivity

The need for services to be 'culturally sensitive' is widely acknowledged, but there are a wide variety of practices and policies that evoke different interpretations of the term. Different levels of cultural sensitivity can be discerned and these relate to various other aspects of good practice. For example, at one level, cultural sensitivity relates to understanding culture as a kind of 'fog' or 'mask' that may obscure aspects of childhood that are assumed to be universal. This is an orientation similar to that of the clinician who tries to detect the prevalence of universal diseases in culturally diverse populations. The anthropologist Aiwa Ong, for example, describes a scenario in a mental health clinic in San Francisco where the function of cultural expertise is to help the psychiatrist reach a diagnosis with Cambodian patients. A cultural mediator is employed to 'translate' the culturally specific symptoms into Western scientific categories to aid psychiatric diagnosis (Ong, 1995). This approach echoes earlier writing on transcultural psychiatry where, for example, Rack describes 'cultural pitfalls' in the recognition of certain psychiatric conditions and cultural knowledge as a key to helping clinicians see through the cultural layers to a 'real' disease entity (Rack, 1982). Processes in which Western psychiatric categories as described in standard diagnostic manuals are applied to culturally diverse groups have been described as based on a 'category fallacy'. Kleinman has argued that 'applying such categories in non-western cultures leads to a category fallacy because by definition it will find what is universal and it will systematically miss what does not fit in tight parameters'

(Kleinman, 1977). He goes on to argue that what is missed is more interesting when one does cross-cultural psychiatry because the missed symptoms will be the most striking examples of the influence of culture on depression.

Kleinman's influential approach to cultural sensitivity may be characterised as drawing the clinical gaze back to encompass a wider field of vision in which the social and cultural worlds of patients and clients are revealed. The concerns of clinicians here are not limited to the identification and treatment of universal disease entities, but encompass the 'explanatory models' of patients and clients themselves. These models are elicited from patients' illness narratives not only to enhance greater understanding between clinicians and patients, but also to actively inform programmes of treatment. As Kleinman argues,

> one of the core tasks in effective clinical care... – one whose value it is all too easy to underrate – is to affirm the patients experience of illness as constituted by lay explanatory models and to negotiate, using the specific terms of those models, an acceptable therapeutic approach.
>
> (Kleinman, 1988, p49)

In addition, a core task for the clinician is 'the empathetic interpretation of a life story that makes over the illness into the subject matter of a biography' (ibid.). What Kleinman refers to as the 'illness narratives', draw on cultural models for arranging experiences and for communicating these experiences. He presents the narratives as not only reflecting illness experience but also as constituting them, arguing that 'over the long course of a disorder, these model texts shape and even create experience' (ibid.).

While Kleinman was not writing here about refugee children, the principles of this approach have been influential in academic literature and educational programmes on refugees and refugee children (Eastmond, 2000). These principles reflect those outlined above in relation to participatory methods in that the approach involves attempting to understand the world from the point of view of those who are the recipients of programmes. It implies further that this engagement and understanding informs the modus operandi of services through the employment of concepts and methods deriving from refugees themselves. This is not to imply that those who adopt a culturally sensitive approach dispense with the knowledge and experience they have derived from their own professional training. The approach suggested here is rather one in which the development of skills in culturally sensitive methods of this kind are integral parts of training for those working with refugee children. A critical reflexivity is developed in which the cultural influences on both the perspectives of professionals and clients are examined. As a number of scholars and practitioners have pointed out, this is not to imply a position of cultural relativism in the sense that any perspective deriving from a cultural context is as valid as any other (Oloyede, 2002; Aroian, 2005). It is rather to suggest that professional knowledge and training is augmented and informed by ongoing scrutiny of the cultural contexts of care.

The application of cultural sensitivity in the reflexive sense described here suggests a movement from a casual utilising of concepts that are routinely applied to refugee children in immigration and welfare contexts, towards a critical scrutiny of the concepts themselves. It suggests an epistemological 'break' of the kind described by Bourdieu, involving questioning of the 'presuppositions inherent in the position of an outside observer' (Bourdieu, 1977, p2). It is, as Barnard observed, 'achieved by subjecting the *position* of the observer to the same critical analysis as that of the constructed object at hand' (cited in Wacquant, 1992, p41, emphasis in original). In the present context, the 'observer' refers not only to researchers involved in the field but also to practitioners whose work involves the construction of refugee children as an objective group of clients requiring intervention from services.

As such, the approach is not only relevant for researchers removed from the day-to-day world of working with refugees, but also one that is vital for practitioners seeking to provide services that are closely attuned to refugees' needs. To take one example from material examined above, in the 'Safe Case Transfer' process in which refugee children were moved from the south east of England, practice was framed from a perspective of cultural appropriateness. This involved a homogenising of the refugee children and their needs according to a rationality which accorded significance to their identities as 'Muslims' or 'Afghans'. A reflexive approach would suggest a critical scrutiny of the categories used to underpin and generate practices leading to a discovery of an engagement with those categories that were salient to the refugee children themselves.

A further and related concern is the extent to which refugees may be routinely perceived as culturally 'embedded'. By this, I refer to the tendency whereby they are viewed, implicitly or explicitly, as mere products of a particular 'culture'. On the basis of this perspective, various kinds of informal and formal 'knowledge' are developed, often reinforcing what are little more than crude stereotypes. Thus, Roma children are viewed as having certain essentialised characteristics as are Congolese, Nigerians, Chechnyans, Somalis and so on. This is not to suggest that generalised statements may never be made, but these should be carefully constructed to reflect salient empirical realities. Furthermore, there is a related tendency to 'blame the culture' in strategic manoeuvres that obscure the impact of racism and the impact of punitive immigration and welfare policies. Fassin has, for example, noted that fires occurring in flats occupied by immigrants in Paris were blamed by authorities on culturally specific cookery techniques rather than on the effect of poor infrastructure and the negligence of landlords. Again, in relation to the health impact of old lead piping Fassin notes how:

> Although the history of childhood lead poisoning started a century ago in the United States, the first French cases were identified in 1985. Instead of merely adopting knowledge accumulated for decades, the public health professionals and activists involved had to reestablish, against incredulity from medical authorities and resistance from policymakers, all the evidence: that children were the main group concerned; that cases were not isolated but part

of an epidemic; that wall paint in old, dilapidated apartments was the source of contamination; and that poor housing conditions, and not cultural practices, were responsible for the high incidence in African families.

(Fassin and Naude, 2004)

Fassin thus draws attention to the role of the cultural in obscuring the social and structural influences on poor health among migrant children. This shifting of emphasis is, I would suggest, not confined to a few instances and localities, but is found frequently within the responses of agencies to refugees and other migrants. 'Blaming the culture' is tantamount to blaming the people themselves and is present in numerous informal and formal comments on parenting, devitalisation, educational achievement, illness, personal hygiene and so on in relation to refugees and refugee children.

Refugee children are seen as culturally embedded in a further and more benign sense, alluded to above. Loss of culture is routinely seen as one of the tragic consequences of forced migration and programmes often seek to offer a culturally appropriate environment to provide a little compensation for this loss. The loss of culture is frequently cited as a contributory factor in poor mental well-being and in the ongoing personal and social difficulties refugees face. While there is certainly much truth in this view, Rapport has argued that agencies should recognise that for many, even forced migrants, displacement can be liberating (Rapport, 2006). It can represent an opportunity to step outside routine constraints of culture and custom and to generate a new sense of identity. This is an important insight and challenges many taken-for-granted views of refugees. For groups that have been oppressed in their countries of origin owing to gender, sexual orientation, ethnicity and other factors, it is certainly possible that some will be more than happy to leave behind aspects of their previous existence. They may also be perplexed at measures taken in host societies to reacquaint them with aspects of the cultures they have left behind. That free-floating cosmopolitanism is often heavily dependent on structural factors such as class and income, should not obscure the fact that many forced migrants do share aspirations to inhabit different cultural worlds. The central point here, and in general in relation to cultural appropriateness, is that refugee children themselves should have a central role in constructing and defining their cultural worlds. It is an ongoing challenge to institutions to address the complexity and fluidity this entails through offering services that are receptive to them.

Evaluation

The final component of good practice proposed here is evaluation. Ostensibly evaluation should be undertaken to inform decisions about a course of actions but wider factors may affect its nature and scope. Central questions include the extent to which evaluation is an integral feature of projects for refugee children, how it is undertaken and what role it has in the ongoing development of projects. A further consideration is the extent to which evaluation is independent, both in the data that may be gathered and in the presentation of results. In outlining the results of two studies of programmes for young asylum seekers in the Netherlands, Ingleby identifies three main types of evaluation. *Plan evaluation* relates to questions about whether an activity is a good idea in principle and whether it takes account of knowledge about the activity and target group. *Process evaluation* relates to what is actually going on in a programme and how it relates to what was intended. *Outcome* (or effect) *evaluation* asks whether the programme is producing the sort of effects that were hoped for. Ingleby argues that the latter are difficult to gauge for many programmes offered to asylum seekers as we are here normally dealing with 'complex activities and subtle effects' (Ingleby, 2005a, p176). Plan evaluation as outlined here may be viewed in other terms as preliminary investigation of the phenomenon in question to arrive at criteria that may be used as evaluative yardsticks. As Milne has observed, 'without clearly defined goals a programme simply cannot be evaluated. It is meaningless to ask the basic evaluative research questions (e.g. "did the programme work"?) without some predetermined objective in mind' (Milne, 1987, p23). Thus investigation of conditions at any site where refugees are based may be used to identify needs and formulate criteria for evaluating a programme. The process evaluation can be seen as a complementary second phase of evaluation and centres on examining the actual activities that are undertaken through a particular programme.

Both the plan and process evaluation may be seen as intrinsic to a programme in that the criteria and methods are grounded in the nature of the activities themselves and involve investigative fieldwork employing qualitative research methods. Effect evaluation suggests the importation of external tools for measurement typically involving some form of rating scales. One basic design is a 'before and after' study to assess, for example, whether there is measurable psychological change in the group. The introduction of a control group helps to ensure the change can be ascribed to the programme itself rather than to some other influence.

Other useful conceptual and methodological distinctions can be drawn between formative and summative evaluation. Formative evaluation relates to an ongoing evaluative process that informs the development of a programme. It involves the production of findings that are studied and discussed and, where deemed appropriate, used to modify the programme. As such, it suggests an evaluative culture that is intrinsic to the organisation. Summative evaluation has some features in common with effect evaluation in that it suggests the role of external experts undertaking a relatively tightly defined study over a prescribed time period. It is summative in the sense that it produces evidence of the overall effect of the programme and normally produces results following the conclusion of a programme or a distinct phase of it.

Put very simply, evaluation refers to the process of assessing the value of a programme or project. This value can be assessed internally in relation to the aims and objectives of the project and externally by standards of care judged acceptable by national and international standards. There is, of course, a significant interrelationship between these two components, as local project standards will be informed by wider national and international standards and conventions.

In formulating evaluative questions it is important to recognise the wider political context in which evaluation studies are commissioned and their results are received. These can be influenced by a concern to delay decision making on particular projects or to deflect criticism for an aspect of the provision of services. Those commissioning studies may have a preconceived notion of what the study should contain and what areas it should not cover and they may be reluctant to support work that does not accord with these preconceptions. In order to ensure that evaluation studies encompass broader political factors, it is appropriate that they encompass the macro, meso and micro framework described above.

In illustrating some of the methodological features of an evaluation involving refugee children, I draw on my evaluation of the Safe Case Transfer project described in Chapter 4. As noted, this centred on the transfer of asylum-seeking children from the south east of England to Manchester and surrounding areas. For the purposes of this study, the macro, meso and micro aspects were distinguished as follows:

Macro level

These related to international and national instruments and agreements, including the UN Convention on the Rights of the Child, the Universal Declaration on Human Rights, the UN Convention on Refugees and national instruments such as the Children Act 1989 and the Hillingdon Judgement.

Meso level

These related to frameworks and guidance linked to the above laws and conventions, including relevant local authority circulars and frameworks outlining good practice in the field.

Micro level

These aspects related to local level agreed operational criteria and its implementation 'on the ground'.

All of the above levels of analysis were incorporated in the study and they provided a reference point in developing case studies, interviews, documentary research and observations. The evaluation examined the processes through which a macro level of national and international guidelines were incorporated into local practices and informed the ongoing development of the project. As noted above, an essential component of evaluation was the assessment of programmes against accepted criteria. The research examined the project against the following elements:

Criterion 1: international guidelines outlined in the Separated Children in Europe programme

A useful framework for the identification of good practice was provided by Save the Children. This incorporates guidelines on good practice from a number of international sources outlined in the vision underpinning the Separated Children in Europe programme. According to the programme guidelines, separated children should:

- feel safe, secure and loved
- have a responsible, trained and independent guardian to whom they may turn
- receive accurate advice, appropriate guidance and support throughout their time in the country of destination
- be seen as a child first and foremost rather than simply a migrant (or criminal) subject to administrative and immigration control
- be seen as a unique individual
- be listened to with respect and be involved in the design of procedures and services addressing their needs
- have their experiences acknowledged and validated
- have opportunities to achieve their full potential
- have their rights protected and realised
- have all their needs – social, emotional and developmental – addressed in relation to each other and not in isolation.

(Save the Children, 2000)

Criterion 2: national criteria

This includes the common features identified as applying to 'Children in Special Circumstances' as outlined in the Framework for the Assessment of Children in Need and their Families (Department of Health, 2000)

Criterion 3: a specific evaluation matrix drawn up for the purposes of the study

This covered six 'domains' identified through consultation with stakeholders and specific questions to investigate the project's performance in relation to the following domains:

Procedures

- How were the procedures drawn up? What criteria were used?
- How do the procedures accord with local, national and international policies and conventions?
- If there are discrepancies, what are the reasons for these?
- Do the procedures form a coherent whole? If not, where are the gaps?

Communication

- Are stakeholders (this category includes refugee children themselves) familiar with the procedures?
- How have they been communicated to them?
- Do they have an opportunity to provide ongoing feedback on the procedures?
- Have users of the service been informed about procedures? If so, how has this been done?
- Do users have an opportunity to provide ongoing feedback?

Comprehension

- Do refugee children and stakeholders understand the aims and objectives of the project?
- Do they understand the procedures?
- Have the procedures been communicated to users in appropriate ways (e.g. jargon free, culturally appropriate)?
- Do stakeholders have a complementary understanding of the procedures?

Implementation

- What steps have been taken to implement the procedures in ongoing practice?
- What problems have been encountered in implementation?
- How have these been addressed?
- Have solutions been found that are satisfactory to refugee children and service providers?

Monitoring

- How are you monitoring the pilot project?
- To what extent are stakeholders, including refugee children, involved in the process?
- Are there gaps in the monitoring?
- How does monitoring data inform the ongoing development of the project?

Dissemination

- How is the experience of the project being recorded?
- How are the results of the project being disseminated among stakeholders?
- Are there mechanisms for receiving feedback and how will this influence future development?
- How are results being disseminated to other authorities?

This is, of course only one example of methodological considerations, criteria and tools that have been used to undertake an evaluation of a programme for refugee children. Relevant criteria and tools will vary depending on the type of evaluation that is undertaken and the practical constraints that may be present. In general terms it may be argued that an essential component is a preliminary phase in which the objectives of the programme are clarified. These should have at least two components; determining objectives from the perspective of the concerns of refugee children themselves and secondly, determining objectives from the perspectives of other stakeholders. A further step is to locate the programme in its institutional context. This can be examined through seeking responses to questions such as 'Who is funding the programme? Why are they funding it?' Furthermore, 'Who is funding the evaluation? And why are they funding it? What purpose will the evaluation have? How will the results be disseminated?' Seeking an early resolution to these questions can help the evaluator to develop a sense of the macro context in which the programme operates. It also could help to reveal the extent to which the evaluation itself is likely to prove influential in the further development of the service. The meso and micro levels at which programmes for refugee children function are significantly influenced by the political and economic contexts in which they operate. It is the task of the evaluation to examine and promote awareness of the interrelationships between these three levels.

On the transfer of good practice

The identification of good practice is not of course simply a method of conferring merit on particular services, but is aimed towards a reproduction of these practices in different localities. In an extensive report into good practice in the mental health and social care of refugees in Europe, salient issues in the transfer of good practice between countries were identified (Watters *et al.*, 2003). These included the production of a standardised template for the examination of services in different countries and locating these within a wider context of policies towards migrants and refugees and the organisation of services. These were important in identifying factors that may inhibit or facilitate the transfer of services between countries. The standardised template for each country included elaboration on the following dimensions:

Demographic data

• immigration and emigration in historical context
• post-World War Two migration: the main groups of immigrants

Political context

• immigration policy; the politics of immigration: public attitudes and media representations
• development of asylum policies, public attitudes and the representation of asylum seekers and refugees in the media

- current admission policies
- current reception and accommodation arrangements
- rights and restrictions applying to asylum seekers (e.g. work, education)
- evidence of the specific challenges faced by asylum seekers and refugees derived from official and professional views; perspectives from the groups themselves; using published research; interview with group members and other informants.

Health and social care provision

- a short overview of the health and social care system in each country
- an overview of multicultural care – including, for example, addressing questions about the extent to which efforts have been made to improve the care of members of ethnic minorities in general; the state of the art in multicultural service provision
- an overview of services for asylum seekers and refugees – including questions regarding what sort of care asylum seekers and refugees are *entitled* to. How *accessible* are these services? What problems have arisen in service provision?

Services developed for asylum seekers and refugees

The approaches developed in each country were categorised under the following headings:

- organisational changes – introduced to improve service provision for asylum seekers and refugees
- training and education
- treatment
- preventive activities.

Good practices

- summary of strong and weak points in service provision
- case studies of good practices – highlighting individual projects or approaches that are felt to be particularly innovative and promising.

Transferring good practices

On the basis of the above identification study the following processes were undertaken towards the transfer of good practice from one country to another:

1   An evaluation was undertaken with selected practices based on existing reports, supplemented where necessary by interviews with professionals and clients who had been involved.

2   Identification of the differences in the parameters of service provision and national context between the countries that may make modification necessary (e.g. differences in the refugee populations, financing of services, structure of service provision, treatment philosophy etc.).

3   Development of proposals regarding the necessary modifications to make practices transferable.

4   Production of manual summarising points 1 to 3 and submitted this to selected experts familiar with the interventions for critical assessment and feedback.

5   Expert meetings were held with key stakeholders in the country to which the intervention was to be transferred, to discuss the best strategy for implementing it.

6   A research team in the country then developed a strategy for implementation and proceeded with piloting and evaluation.

7   Finally, the success of the transfer was evaluated and recommendations made about continuation or modification of the innovation.

(adapted from Watters *et al.*, 2003)

This template and methodology was developed in the context of a study of good practice in the mental health and social care of asylum seekers and refugees, which drew particularly on studies in four European countries – the UK, the Netherlands, Spain and Portugal, but also included smaller scale studies in Canada, Australia and Guatemala (Watters *et al.*, 2003). While the approach described here was directed towards asylum seekers and refugees, its components would be similarly helpful in the identification and dissemination of good practices towards refugee children. It could also provide a useful framework for undertaking studies of the transferability of good practices within a country. In this instance some of the broad contextual aspects could be modified to take account of similarities in the political and policy environments.

To briefly illustrate two examples from the 2003 study, the transfer of schools-based programmes for refugee children in the Netherlands to the UK was complicated owing to the fact that the children in the Netherlands were largely taught in reception centres outside of mainstream provision. In transferring the initiative to the UK, it was adapted to the delivery of the programme to refugee children in mainstream schools and was subsequently formally introduced into schools in the Manchester area with support from the Ethnic Minority Achievement Grant (see p117). In another example, the model of a specialist mental health team for refugees in the UK was considered in terms of transfer to the Netherlands. The team operated a low threshold, culturally sensitive, 'one-stop' service offering counselling and support and referring those in need to appropriate mental health or social care agencies. As in the example of the Dutch schools programme, a manual was developed for consideration by a team of experts who considered the feasibility of incorporation into the other country. While the latter programme was viewed as having many merits and suitable for some sections of the Dutch refugee population, its implementation was dependent on support from Dutch mental health service providers who would be prepared to bid for funding to take matters forward. In the event, owing to financial constraints and a declining population of asylum seekers, no agency in the Netherlands was willing to support the transfer (Watters and Ingleby, 2004).

The basic principle here is that practices are developed and sustained in specific institutional and service contexts and underpinned by distinctive professional perspectives on care. In seeking to achieve the transfer of good practice, it is important first to be satisfied that the initiative in question fulfils explicit and robust criteria for good practice. Second, the service should be located within its broader context, incorporating what has been described here as both an immigration and a welfare trajectory. Finally, transfer is dependent on introduction into a new environment and it is vital to engage with local experts to assess the feasibility of its incorporation in a new institutional and service context (Watters and Ingleby, 2004).

Conclusion

What was outlined above are six dimensions of good practice in programmes for refugee children that can be used as a framework for investigating a wide range of programmes that have been developed for this group. These dimensions reflect overarching themes that have been identified in this book, including the importance of recognising children's agency, the need to examine the political and socio-economic contexts in which refugee children emerge and are placed, the importance of examining the moral economy of care and the discursive formations within which refugee children become embedded. Those working with refugee children are often doing so within a broad climate of suspicion and increasingly controlled and restrictive services. In this context good practices are often produced by committed professionals who are astute in navigating a complex and rapidly changing environment. Within this environment the dimensions of good practices identified above may be most appropriately seen as linked to a series of 'accomplishments' achieved through a combination of innovation, flexibility and commitment. These accomplishments will be outlined in the following chapter.

8　Conclusion
Seven accomplishments in the care of refugee children

Drawing on the evidence presented here of the ways in which refugee children are treated in a variety of potential 'host' countries, two broad strategies can be discerned. I characterise these as strategies of non-incorporation and biolegitimacy, respectively. In the first strategy the orientation may be characterised as non-incorporation or deflection. Here it is not so much a question of offering children poor treatment as of *preventing children being incorporated into distinctive politico-legal spaces* where claims of asylum may be made and legally required welfare support provided. The strategy of non-incorporation underpins a raft of measures directed towards repelling children without proper entry documents from entering countries, or for removing them swiftly if they have.

These include stringent border controls, for example, the introduction of juxtaposed controls whereby the processing of potential immigrants takes place outside of a potential country of destination. The strategy of non-incorporation also governs some practices noted in the southern Mediterranean region, whereby potential asylum seekers have been forcibly removed from border areas and driven to locations deep inside the territories they are trying to pass through. It has also been noted as manifest in the absence of advice and resources necessary to initiate asylum claims in many of the reception areas. In the case of Zeebrugge in Belgium, non-incorporation is reflected in the 'light-touch' adopted by the authorities towards the children they apprehended trying to pass through the port hidden in lorries. The minimal procedures adopted deterred children from claiming asylum with all its legal and welfare implications and indirectly encouraged continued attempts to reach the UK. Similar considerations can be seen as underpinning the return of apprehended children found by border patrol officers in the US. In a telling phrase, Bhabha and Crock note that, 'the children these officials meet are often physically located on US territory, but not considered legally "present"' (Bhabha and Crock, 2007, p34). They note that some of those who do not have valid visas will be turned away immediately before ever being admitted to the country, while others will be given an option of voluntary return as an alternative to appearing in court.

The strategy of non-incorporation is not as such governed by passivity but by calculated and active strategies that effectively place asylum off the agenda. I have earlier associated this with Lukes' analysis of power, specifically the 'two-dimensional view' involving the examination of the mechanisms whereby power is exercised by ensuring certain items are kept off agendas (Lukes, 2005). Non-incorporation is also appropriately considered in relation to a 'state of exception' in which guarantees of legal protection and entitlement are circumscribed or suspended (Agamben, 2005). In examining the historical and philosophical contexts in which states of exception arise, Agamben notes its recurrent justification through a concept of necessity in which '"necessity has no law" which is interpreted in two opposing ways: "necessity does not recognise any law" and "necessity creates its own law"' (2005, p24). The myriad strategies and processes recorded by human rights bodies such as Amnesty International and Human Rights Watch reflect contexts in which the activity of officials appears governed by an overriding view of a state of necessity.

The modus operandi here recalls Judith Butler's reflection that a state of emergency shifts the operation of power from a set of laws to a set of rules. The latter are 'not binding by virtue of established law or modes of legitimation, but fully discretionary, even arbitrary, wielded by officials who interpret them unilaterally and decide the condition and form of their invocation' (Butler, 2004, p62). This observation, made in the context of a paper on the introduction of indefinite detention following 9/11, is also telling in relation to the various micro processes operating in border areas and reception centres. However, while a good deal of localised discretion may be at play in invoking and implementing rules, these are here governed by the overriding objective of deterrence. As Bhabha and colleagues have noted, children, like other migrants, are entitled to apply for asylum without any prior permission or legal processing. While their application is pending, removal is prohibited. However, to apply for asylum, 'children – like all other asylum seekers – have to get access to the country in the first place' (Bhabha and Crock, 2007, p141).

The prevention of would-be asylum seekers from entering a territory is achieved by a range of measures including non-entrée, interdiction and offshore processing. Besides the juxtaposed controls referred to above, non-entrée measures include the tightening of visa restrictions on nationals of visa-producing countries and the imposition of severe fines on transport companies operating airlines, ships, trains or lorries that have been used to transport undocumented migrants. The measures also include increasing surveillance and the introduction of airline liaison officers to provide additional documentation checks before passengers travel. The strategy is supported by a range of bi-lateral and international agreements aimed at supporting border control in intermediate countries that would-be asylum seekers travel through en route. It is not only the country on the immediate border that is an object of deterrence measures, but also those countries in proximity to it. The US, for example, supports Mexico to patrol its southern border and deport people from other Latin American countries before they travel further north (Bhabha and Crock, 2007, p142). Inda notes that since 9/11 concerns have also been raised that the US southern border is being crossed by would-be terrorists from beyond Latin America, leading to a raft of new policies of deterrence (2006, p119).

Further strategies of non-incorporation include the determination that certain countries of origin are safe and that nationals from these countries could be dealt with by fast-track procedures. Indeed, in the case of Australia, Bhabha and Crock note that its laws 'now include provisions that bar applications from individuals travelling from certain countries' and limitations on protection obligations in respect of any person who spends seven days or more in a country where he or she could have sought protection from either the state or the offices of UNHCR (2007, p143). Restrictions on applications from certain countries have been introduced in many countries despite UNHCR guidance that 'stresses that claims should be considered on their individual merits, not by blanket assessments of the general situation in countries of origin' (UNHCR, 1992). The UK, for example, introduced a so-called 'White List' of countries in 1996 that were deemed to have no general risk of persecution. Those who were determined to be from these countries were subject to a fast-track procedure that reduced the likelihood of their claim being accepted. It has been noted that although the list was abolished in 1999, a variant was reintroduced in 2002, 'initially involving prospective new EU Member States, but extended in 2003 to involve other countries including, astonishingly, Sri Lanka' (Good, 2007, p102).

Further measures that may be subsumed under the heading of non-incorporation include the interdiction of migrants, normally at sea, and the creation of offshore centres for processing their applications. This practice has been associated in particular with Australia where a number of researchers have noted evidence of some particularly draconian approaches. Bhabha and Crock, for example, observe that 'initiatives were taken in Indonesia to sabotage boats that were to carry asylum seekers to Australia, forcing them to abort their illicit journey' (2007, p143). Moorehead has recounted the story of the 'Tampa', a Norwegian cargo ship that rescued a sinking boat carrying 438 asylum seekers heading from Indonesia towards the Australian territory of Christmas Island. Despite their pleas, and in the face of considerable political manoeuvrings, the Australian government resisted requests for the people to land on Australian soil.

This event was a precursor to the introduction of systematic processes of offshore processing in which territories owned by Australia and which had been used as dropping off points for asylum seekers 'were "excised" by Australia for the purposes of migration' (Moorehead, 2005, p108). Moorehead describes the process initiated in 2001 as follows;

> all future boatloads of illegal people would not be allowed...to reach Australia. They would, if possible, be intercepted at sea and returned to Indonesia. If not, they would be transferred to offshore processing centres and to a number of designated countries willing to hold them in detention while their futures were sorted out. At no time would they have access to Australia's legal processes and there would be no right of appeal.
>
> (Moorehead, 2005, p108)

Children have not been excluded from these processes and indeed have been routinely the subjects of mandatory detention and offshore processing. Processes of interdiction have also been noted in the US with only a 'tiny number of intercepted migrants escaping return to their country of origin'. They are usually returned to their port of embarkation or sent to 'Guantanamo Bay in Cuba for refugee processing and (if successful), resettlement in a third country' (Bhabha and Crock, 2007, p144).

The Committee on the Rights of the Child which monitors the Convention on the Rights of the Child has criticised measures 'to artificially exclude some parts of a territory from the reach of domestic law', as these violate states' international obligations. The committee argues that 'state obligations cannot be arbitrarily and unilaterally curtailed either by excluding zones or areas from a state's territory or by defining particular zones or areas as not, or only partly, under the jurisdiction of the state' (ibid., p144). Bhabha and Crock have argued that besides fundamental humanitarian concerns with respect to the processes involved in offshore processing, there are notable differences for children in terms of the acceptance rates for asylum claims. They note that of 55 children sent to the island of Nauru for processing in 2002–03, 32 young Afghans were returned to their country while no child was returned to Afghanistan having been through the legal processes in mainland Australia (ibid., p150). They also note that while non-entrée and interdiction policies have an adversarial impact on all asylum seekers, their effect is particularly acute for unaccompanied or separated children, 'without resources to demand a hearing, to make safe arrangements, or to provide evidence in support of their claim for protection'. Introduction policies also violate international law by 'denying child asylum seekers the right to seek asylum and protection and *refoulement* to their countries; compromising their rights to liberty, security, and protection of their best interests; and violating their basic claims to humanitarian care' (ibid., p144).

As we have noted, when children enter the asylum system, no matter how poorly it may be administered, it is at considerable cost, directly or indirectly, to governments. A strategy of non-incorporation is not confined to processes of deterring would-be asylum seekers, but can also be seen in many of the policies and practices introduced for children following their asylum application. Here it applies to the broadly defined area of social care, encompassing rules governing access areas such as education, accommodation, health care and legal support. In Denmark, for example, this non-incorporation is reinforced through the contracting out of all aspects of care to a third party – the Red Cross. In many of the examples given above, children are placed in a marginal position in relation to mainstream services; receiving education and health services in reception centres or being placed in detention.

The second strategy identified here is biolegitimacy. This concept was evoked in Fassin's observations on the situation of undocumented migrants in France at the end of the 1990s. He documented a striking statistical correlation between sharply declining rates of acceptance of claims for asylum, accompanied by a concomitant increase in numbers of claimants who were allowed to remain in the country on humanitarian grounds, often on the basis of ill health. As noted, Fassin argued that while these figures indicated increasing scepticism towards claims of persecution on political grounds, they indicated a form of legitimacy based on the sick body (Fassin, 2001). While Fassin's papers have not focused particularly on refugee children, the central concept of biolegitimacy has significant resonance in this field, albeit with some qualification.

We have noted above that refugee children are routinely embedded in discourses of trauma, vulnerability, socio-emotional problems and risk. These underpin a large number of the totality of programmes offered for refugee children, for example the various schools programmes centred around processes of social and emotional rehabilitation. Participation in these programmes and, by extension, in these discourses provides an avenue of legitimacy wherein refugee children are given social recognition and professional support on the basis of their perceived problems. This is often within contexts of widespread public scepticism and hostility towards asylum seekers in general. While it is certainly the case that a number of refugee children experience conditions such as PTSD and various emotional problems and may benefit from professional interventions, accounting for the ubiquity of this orientation requires more than clinical considerations. Kleinman *et al.* have noted the role played by political and professional processes in 'powerfully shaping the responses to types of social suffering'. These include authorised and contested appropriations of collective suffering – a central aspect of which is medicalisation. 'The state, its institutions, and groups that contest state control press medicalization for its advantages in regulating persons, their bodies, and networks' (1997, pxii). Arguably the placing of refugee children within programmes where their suffering is rendered professionally intelligible and managed allows them a position within a preordained social system. Summerfield, for one, has cautioned against this approach arguing that 'there may be risks that the host society offers refugees a sick role rather than what is really sought: opportunities for meaningful citizenship as part of rebuilding a way of life' (2005, p111).

As Kleinman implies, an orientation towards medicalisation is not only promoted through the state and its institutions, but may be constitutive of oppositional strategies. In Australia, a team of mental health experts led by the psychiatrist Derrick Silove campaigned effectively against processes of mandatory detention by documenting its negative impact on aggravating or causing mental health problems. According to Moorehead's account,

> Using a wide battery of internationally accepted tests and criteria, the doctors found that a third of the adults had resorted to some form of self-harm; that every adult could be diagnosed as suffering from a depressive disorder; that all the children showed signs of at least one psychiatric disorder and 86 per cent of them had multiple disorders.
>
> (2005, p119)

A range of concerns on the impact of mandatory detention on children's wellbeing resulted in a large-scale government inquiry into children in immigration detention by the Human Rights and Equal Opportunity Commission. A substantial part of the commission's report focused on the mental health implications of detention where the following observations were made:

The Alliance of Health Professionals, which includes a majority of the medical colleges in Australia, suggested that: 'Current practices of detention of infants and children are likely to have both immediate and longer-term effects on children's development, psychological and emotional health'.[4]

More specifically, evidence provided to the Inquiry by children and their families, detention centre medical staff, consultant psychiatrists as well as psychiatric studies on children in detention indicate that a range of factors contribute to the presence of psychological problems in children in immigration detention. Those factors include one or more of:

- torture and trauma prior to arrival in Australia
- the length of detention
- uncertainty as to the visa process and negative visa decisions
- the breakdown of many families within detention
- living in a closed environment
- children's perception that they are not safe within detention
- treatment of children by detention staff.

A conclusion drawn on the basis of this evidence was as follows: 'the cases and situations described in this chapter demonstrate the connection between long-term detention and the declining psychological health of certain children and this alone is sufficient to find a breach of international law' (Human Rights and Equal Opportunity Commission, 2004).

The legitimacy here does not emerge directly from the condition of the children but from the investigation and representation of suffering through clinical scales and psychiatric diagnosis. These findings are lent further credibility by the authoritative endorsement of formal health professional bodies and medical colleges. The example is one of strategic categorisation in the sense that the problems of refugees are rendered both intelligible and legitimate through their position within socially sanctioned and officially supported discourses (Watters, 2001a). The findings here have the weight of medical science behind them and this is a powerful influence in changing official and public attitudes.

The oppositional role of biolegitimacy is arguably also evidenced through the phenomenon of severe withdrawal behaviour, discussed in Chapter 5. Here the question of legitimacy remains indeterminate. The children's condition has not been recognised as according with any clearly demarcated psychiatric diagnosis and their credibility remains under question by official bodies. The very title employed by the authorities – 'severe withdrawal behaviour' – is suggestive of uncertainties with respect to clinical authenticity and aetiology. Arguably, the condition may be seen as an attempt by the asylum seekers themselves to achieve biolegitimacy by representing their suffering through the sick bodies of children. As such it is a call for clinical attention and the allegiance of the doctor in a context where other avenues of legitimacy are seen as failing. The phenomenon may thus be seen as an example of strategic categorisation, only here initiated by asylum seekers themselves.

The two broad strategies identified here are underpinned by specific views of the refugee child, suggesting an addition to earlier sociological formulations (James *et al.*, 1998). Based on the strategies of non-incorporation and biolegitimacy, refugee children are seen as being one of two types; the *untrustworthy child* and the *damaged child*. The former has no claim for legitimacy and should be deflected from the territory, while the latter has legitimacy only by virtue of a damaged psychological and emotional condition. The strategies and orientations that underpin these views are outlined in Table 8.1.

These strategies are supported by particular political orientations. Non-incorporation is governed by states of exception and necessity in which perceived threats of a mass influx of migrants from poorer countries leads to the introduction of specific rules aimed at deterrence. As noted, the strategy may be seen also as operating in respect of asylum seekers who have managed to make claims on a territory through a raft of processes and procedures that keep them in marginalised positions. The desired position of 'host' countries appears to be one in which asylum seekers go through necessary procedures with a minimal impingement on host societies' social care institutions. To coin a phrase adopted for a study of British immigration controls, asylum seekers can be seen as such as being 'governed at a distance' (Morris, 1998). Strategies of non-incorporation are linked to an emphasis on refugee children as being untrustworthy. This perspective underpins the routine official scepticism accorded to their claims for asylum, their age and their personal histories. As Nadine Finch, a barrister working with child asylum seekers, has argued in her extensive study of the UK system:

> There appears to be an almost universal culture of disbelief within the Immigration and Nationality Directorate in relation to asylum applications from unaccompanied or separated children and there is no evidence of a liberal application of the benefit of the doubt to children's applications. For example, trafficked children and child soldiers are regularly refused asylum on the basis that their accounts of persecution are unpersuasive even when there is considerable corroborating evidence.
>
> (2005, p194)

This culture of disbelief is reflected in the very low rates of successful asylum applications from children, with Finch noting that in the UK only 2 to 4 per cent of children were granted asylum between 2003 and 2004 (Finch, 2005, p58). In the UK the practice is normally not to return children to their home countries unless there are adequate reception and care arrangements in place there. 'In

Table 8.1

Strategy	View of the refugee child	Political orientation
Non-incorporation	The untrustworthy child	State of exception
Biolegitimacy	The damaged child	Governmentality

practice, no enquiries are usually made about the adequacy of such arrangements, a child is just granted discretionary leave until he or she is eighteen' (ibid.). While this outcome may produce some immediate benefit in that the child is allowed to stay until reaching 18, it does not acknowledge that the child is in any need of protection. Similarly, embedded cultures of disbelief have been identified internationally, affecting all aspects of the asylum determination processes.

While states of exception may be seen as governing the strategies of non-incorporation, a governmentality approach is useful in the examination of processes of biolegitimacy and the attendant emphasis on the sick or damaged child. A broadly conceptualised governmentality approach suggests an investigative and methodological orientation that encompasses the processes whereby refugee children are categorised and embedded in specific discursive formations. Its orientation is towards analysis of the ways in which refugee children *are* incorporated into societies through specific avenues of access and forms of legitimacy. This field of enquiry encompasses forms of incorporation identified by Ong, whereby refugees become 'new kinds of subjects, mastering the codes and rules of bona fide refugees, compliant aid recipients and good patients' (2003, p65).

These orientations provide modes of contextualising the systems of social care that are applied to refugee children. As has been argued throughout, it is vitally important to achieve an understanding of the various initiatives developed for refugee children through placing them within their wider political and institutional contexts. This task is not only theoretical but practical and a vital aspect in the transfer of good practice in this field. The material presented throughout this book identifies various dispositions found in services for refugee children. These are often borne of a priori assumptions about refugee children and their needs and delivered within very restrictive institutional settings.

Attempts to improve services for refugee children must recognise the limitations placed by these contexts but simultaneously be aware of the potential for change and development. Outlined below are seven accomplishments that represent, I believe, realistic goals for the development of services and can form a useful template for undertaking service evaluation. They are informed by the lessons from various research projects on the health and social care of refugee children that underpin the material presented in this book and draw on the discussion of good practice presented above. While suggestive of distinctive aspects of social care practice, the accomplishments represent interrelated and complementary aspects.

The accomplishments are as follows:

1   *Take refugee children seriously as competent interpreters of their own lives.*
    This accomplishment orientates services towards listening and receptivity. This is not to deny that refugee children are often confused and distressed and having difficulties in adapting to a new environment. What it does suggest is that refugee children themselves may be the best resource for seeking an understanding of these problems and challenges and further, that they are not only the subjects of severely adverse circumstances, but are also resourceful and capable in exercising agency. In practical terms this accomplishment suggests

an overall orientation for services for refugee children that can infuse the policies, practices and organisational cultures of service providing agencies.

2   *A holistic approach which offers integrated programmes of social, emotional and psychological support*

The adoption of a holistic approach implies receptivity to refugee children's needs and flexible ways of working that combine counselling, advocacy and interagency work. This model has been adopted in a number of contexts in countries of reception and has received encouraging results from evaluation studies (Watters *et al.*, 2003). Adopting the model has implications for staff training and interprofessional working arrangements.

3   *A receptivity towards culture*

This accomplishment suggests moving from approaches that either ignore refugee children's cultures or treat children as though they were necessarily embedded in one specific culture. As such it is a perspective that moves away from what Sen has defined as 'plural monoculturalism' (Sen, 2006). It suggests receptivity to children's own sense of their culture while recognising that their conceptions may be fluid and display multiple influences.

4   *A recognition of the impact of ongoing events on refugee children's lives*

This accomplishment orientates services towards the here and now of refugee children's lives. This is not to suggest that past events and future orientations are not important for refugee children and should not be worked through in programmes. What it does imply is that the present is a useful starting point for interactions, including an ongoing assessment of factors in the here and now that are impinging on children's lives.

5   *An orientation towards empowerment through ownership and participation*

This accomplishment orients programmes and services towards providing refugee children with a sense of ownership through their active participation in, for example, setting agendas or planning exercises. There is strong evidence to show that a sense of participation and engagement enhances mental well-being. Appropriate levels of participation depend on the context and the capacities of the children.

6   *An engagement with family and meaningful others*

This accomplishment suggests that refugee children's families and friends should have opportunities to be involved in programmes and parents should be consulted with respect to children's participation. This accomplishment will help to avoid the danger of professionals creating 'divided worlds' between children and their families, and offer a sense of continuity and support.

7   *An emphasis on enhancing refugee children's own capabilities*

Sen has pointed out that development has to encompass the task of expanding human capabilities and promoting freedom in a context of social responsibility. He identifies certain 'instrumental freedoms' that have a role in enhancing and guaranteeing the substantive freedoms of individuals (Sen, 1999, pxii). Within the constrained environments experienced by refugee children many of the facilities necessary for enhancing their capabilities may be lacking. The final accomplishment concerns the provision of an appropriate infrastructure that will promote capabilities including educational resources, reasonable accommodation, health care and opportunities for social engagement and play.

These accomplishments are not utopian and many already form a cornerstone of services in reception countries. Many dedicated professionals have developed modes of working with refugee children that are both receptive and participative and which have greatly enhanced children's sense of well-being. What this formulaic presentation may offer is a useful way in which these aspects can be operationalised in the promotion of good practice.

Notes

2 Theoretical orientations

1 It is important to add that this comment is not broadly relevant to the authors' work, which does include substantial consideration of actors' responses to globalisation.

3 Children at borders

2 Said (2000) has pointed out that the phrase is not originally that of Huntington, but of Bernard Lewis.

4 Unaccompanied minors

3 The Queen on the application of B v. London borough of Merton, July 2003.

8 Conclusion

4 See www.hreoc.gov.au/human_rights/children_detention_report/report/

Bibliography

Agamben, G. (1998) *Homo Sacer: Sovereign Power and Bare Life.* Stanford University Press. Stanford, CA.

Agamben, G. (2005) *State of Exception.* University of Chicago Press. Chicago.

Ager, A. (1993) *Mental health issues in refugee populations: a review.* Working paper of the Harvard Center for the Study of Culture and Medicine. Harvard Medical School. Harvard, MA.

Ager, A. and Strang, A. (2004) *Indicators of Integration.* Final report. Home Office. London.

Amit, A. and Rapport, N. (2002) *The Trouble with Community: Anthropological Reflections on Movement, Identity and Collectivity.* Pluto Press. London.

Amnesty International (2005a) *Spain: The Southern Border.* Amnesty International. London.

Amnesty International (2005b) *Italy, Temporary Stay – Permanent Rights: The Treatment of Foreign Nationals Detained in 'Temporary Stay and Assistance Centres' (CPTAs).* Amnesty International. London.

Amnesty International (2005c) *Country Report: Belgium.* Amnesty International. London. http://web.amnesty.org/report2005/bel-summary-eng, accessed 21st September 2006.

Amnesty International (2006) *Italy: Invisible Children – The Human Rights of Migrant and Asylum Seeking Minors Detailed upon Arrival at the Maritime Border in Italy.* Amnesty International. London.

Anderson, P. (2001) 'You don't belong here in Germany...' On the social situation of refugee children in Germany. *Journal of Refugee Studies* 14(2), 187–199.

Ansell, N. (2005) *Children, Youth and Development. Routledge Perspectives on Development.* Routledge. London.

Antoniou, V. and Reynolds, R. (2005) Asylum seeking children in English pre-schools: inclusion and support in the new climate. In Anderssen, H., Ascher, H., Bjornberg, U., Eastmund, M. and Mellander, L. (eds) *The Asylum Seeking Child in Europe.* Centre for European Research at Gothenburg University. Gothenburg.

Apfel, R. and Simon, B. (2000) Mitigating discontents with children in war: an ongoing psychoanalytic inquiry. In Robben, A. and Suarez-Orozco, M. (eds) *Cultures Under Siege: Collective Violence and Trauma.* Cambridge University Press. Cambridge.

Appa, V. (2005) *A Study on how Asylum Seekers and Refugees Access Education in Four Local Authorities in England.* National Children's Bureau. London.

Appadurai, A. (1996) *Modernity at Large: Cultural Dimensions of Globalisation.* Minnesota University Press. Minnesota.

ARC (2002) *Newsletter of the asylum rights campaign* – EU Working Group, September 2002.

Arnot, M. and Pinson, H. (2005) *The Education of Asylum Seeker and Refugee Children: A Study of Local Education Authority and School Values, Policies and Practices.* Faculty of Education, University of Cambridge. Cambridge.

Aroian, K. (2005) Reconciling cultural relativism for a clinical paradigm: what's a nurse to do? *Journal of Professional Nursing* 21(6), 330–331.

Audit Commission (2000) *Another Country: Implementing Dispersal under the Immigration and Asylum Act 1999.* Audit Commission Publications. London.

Ayotte, W. and L. Williamson (2001) *Separated Children in the UK: An Overview of the Current Situation.* Refugee Council and Save the Children. London.

Baldwin, S. (ed.) (1998) *Needs Assessment and Community Care: Clinical Practice and Policy Making.* Butterworth. Heinemann. Oxford.

Balibar, E. (2004) *We the People of Europe: Reflections on Transnational Citizenship.* Princeton University Press. Princeton.

Bartlett, W., Roberts, J. and Le Grand, J. (1998) *A Revolution in Social Policy: Quasi-market Reforms in the 1990s.* Policy Press. Bristol.

Bauer, E. and Thompson, P. (2006) Jamaican mutual aid. In Buonfino, A. and Mulgan, G. (eds) *Porcupines in Winter: The Pleasures and Pains of Living Together in Modern Britain.* The Young Foundation. London.

Bauman, Z. (2004) *Wasted Lives: Modernity and its Outcasts.* Polity. Cambridge.

Benhabib, S. (2002) *The Claims of Culture: Equality and Diversity in the Global Era.* Princeton University Press. Princeton.

Benjamin, W. (1999) Thesis on the philosophy of history. In Benjamin, W. *Illuminations.* Pimlico. London.

Bennaars, G., Seif, H. and Mwangi, D. (1996) *Mid-Decade Review of Progress towards Education for All. The Somalia Case Study.* UNESCO. Nairobi.

Berger, J. (2003) A moment in Ramallah. *London Review of Books*, 24th July.

Berry, J. de, Fazili, A., Farhad, S., Nasiry, F., Hashemi, S. and Hakimi, M. (2003) *The Children of Kabul: Discussions with Afghan Families.* Save the Children. UNICEF.

Bhabha, J. and Crock, M. (2007) *Seeking Asylum Alone: Unaccompanied and Separated Children and Refugee Protection in Australia, the UK and the US.* Themis Press. Sydney.

Bhabha, J. and Finch, N. (2006) *Seeking Asylum Alone: Unaccompanied and Separated Children and Refugee Protection in the UK.* Macarthur Foundation. Cambridge, MA.

Bhabha, J. and Schmidt, S. (2006) *Seeking Asylum Alone: Unaccompanied and Separated Children and Refugee Protection in the United States.* Macarthur Foundation. Cambridge, MA.

Bloom, M. (1990) The psychosocial constructs of social competency. In Gullotta, T.P., Adams, G.R. and Montemayor, R. (eds) *Developing Social Competency in Adolescence*, (pp.11–27). Newbury Park, CA: Sage Publications.

Booth, W. (1994) On the idea of the moral economy. *American Political Science Review* 88(3), 653–667.

Bourdieu, P. (1977) *Outline of a Theory of Practice. Cambridge Studies in Social Anthropology.* Cambridge University Press. Cambridge.

Bourdieu, P. and Passeron, J.-C. (1990) *Reproduction in Education, Society and Culture.* 2nd Edition. Sage. London.

Bourdieu, P. and Wacquant, L. (1992) *An Invitation to Reflexive Sociology.* Polity Press. Cambridge.

Bourdieu, P. and Wacquant, L. (1999) On the cunning of imperialist reason. *Theory, Culture & Society* 16(1), 41–58.

Boyden, J. and de Berry, J. (eds) (2004) *Children and Youth on the Front Line*. Berghahn Books. New York.

Brettell, C. and Hollifield, J. (2000) *Migration Theory: Talking Across Disciplines*. Routledge. New York.

Brown, G. and Harris, T. (1978) *Social Origins of Depression*. Tavistock Publications. London.

Buck-Morss, S. (1977) *The Origin of Negative Dialectics*. The Free Press. New York.

Butler, J. (2004) *Precarious Lives: The Powers of Mourning and Violence*. Verso. London.

Caplan, M.Z. and Weissberg, R.P (1988) Promoting social competence in early adolescence: developmental considerations. In Schneider, G.H., Attili, G., Nadel, J. and Weissberg, R.P. (eds) *Social Competence in Developmental Perspective*, (pp.371–386). Kluwer Academic Publishers. Boston, MA.

Castells, M. (2000) *The Information Age: Economy, Society and Culture*. End of Millennium 2nd Edition. Blackwell. Oxford.

Castles, S. (2003) Towards a sociology of forced migration and social transformation. *Sociology* 37(1), 13–34.

Castles, S. and Miller, M. (2003) *The Age of Migration*. 3rd Edition. Macmillan. Basingstoke.

Castles, S., Crawley, H. and Loughna, S. (2003) *States of Conflict: Causes and Patterns of Forced Migration to the EU and Policy Responses*. Institute of Public Policy Research. London.

Certeau, M. de (1984) *The Practice of Everyday Life*. University of California Press. Berkeley.

Cicchetti, D. (2003) Foreword. In Luthar, S. (ed.) *Resilience and Vulnerability: Adaptation in the Context of Childhood Adversities*. Cambridge University Press. Cambridge.

Clifford, J. (1994) Diasporas. *Cultural Anthropology* 9(3), 302–338.

Coleman, J. (1988) Social capital and the creation of human capital. *American Journal of Sociology* 94, Supplement: S95–S120.

Collyer, M. (2004) *The development impact of temporary international labour migration on southern Mediterranean sending countries: contrasting examples of Morocco and Egypt*. Working paper T6. Development Research Centre on Migration, Globalisation and Poverty. University of Sussex. Brighton.

Cornelius, W. (2004) Spain: the uneasy transition for labor exporter to labor importer. In Cornelius, W., Tsuda, T., Martin, P. and Hollifield, J. (eds) (2004) *Controlling Migration: A Global Perspective*. Stanford University Press. Stanford, CA.

Cornelius, W., Tsuda, T., Martin, P. and Hollifield, J. (eds) (2004) *Controlling Migration: A Global Perspective*. Stanford University Press. Stanford, CA.

Courau, H. (2003) 'Tomorrow Inch Allah, Chance!' *People Smuggler Networks in Sangatte Immigrants and Minorities* 22(2–3), 374–387. Routledge. London.

Crawley, H. (2006) *Child First, Migrant Second: Ensuring that Every Child Matters*. Immigration Law Practitioners Association. London.

Cunningham, R. and Sarayrah, Y. (1993) *Wasta: The Hidden Force in Middle Eastern Society*. Praeger. Westport, CT.

CVS Consultants (1999) *Shattered World: The Mental Health Needs of Refugees and Newly Arrived Communities*. Migrant and Refugees Community Forum and CVS Consultants. London.

Davies, M. and Webb, E. (2000) Promoting the psychological well-being of refugee children. *Clinical Child Psychology and Psychiatry* 5(4), 1359–1045.

Dench, G., Gavron, K. and Young, M. (2006) *The New East End: Kinship, Race and Conflict.* Profile Books. London.

Denoeux, G. (2005) The politics of corruption in Palestine – evidence from recent public opinion poles. *Middle East Policy* 12(3), 119–135.

Department of Health (2000) *Framework for the Assessment of Children in Need and Their Families.* HMSO. Norwich.

Department of Health (2003) Guidance on accommodating children in need and their families. *Local Authority Circular* (2003) 13th June. Department of Health. London.

Derluyn, I. and Broekaert, E. (2005) On the way to a better future: Belgium as a transit country for trafficking and smuggling of unaccompanied minors. *International Migration* 43(4), 31–56.

Doherty, C. (2001) Gardai say stowaways came to Ireland by mistake. *Irish Times*, 11th December.

Dona, G. (2006) Children as research advisors: contributions to a 'methodology of participation' in research children in difficult circumstances. *International Journal of Migration, Health and Social Care* 2(2), 1–15.

Durkheim, E. (1961) *Moral Education.* The Free Press. Glencoe.

Dwivedi, K. (2003) *Meeting the Needs of Ethnic Minority Children: A Handbook for Professionals.* Jessica Kingsley Publishers. London.

Eagleton, T. (1990) *The Ideology of the Aesthetic.* Blackwell Publishing. Oxford.

Eastmond, M. (1998) Nationalist discourses and the construction of difference: Bosnian Muslim refugees in Sweden. *Journal of Refugee Studies* 11(2), 161–181.

Eastmond, M. (2000) Refugees and health: ethnographic approaches. In Ahearn, F. (ed.) *Psychosocial Wellness of Refugees: Issues in Qualitative and Quantitative Research.* Berghahn Books. New York.

Endersby, C. (2007) *Between Risk and Resilience.* Unpublished PhD Thesis. University of Kent. Canterbury.

Esping-Andersen, G. (1990) *The Three Worlds of Welfare Capitalism.* Polity Press. Cambridge.

Essakkili, S. (2007) *Seeking Asylum Alone in the Netherlands.* Vrije Universiteit. Amsterdam.

European Commission (2003) Council Directive 2003/9/EC of 27th January 2003. Laying down minimum standards for the reception of asylum seekers. *Official Journal of the European Union*, L 31.18, 6.2.2003. European Commission. Brussels.

Evans, T. and Harris, J. (2004) Street level bureaucracy, social work and the (exaggerated) death of discretion. *British Journal of Social Work* 34, 871–895.

Eyber, C. and Ager, A. (2004) Researching young people's experiences of war: participatory methods and the trauma discourse in Angola. In Boyden, J. and de Berry, J. (eds) *Children and Youth on the Front Line.* Berghahn Books. New York.

Farmer, P. (1997) On suffering and structural violence. In Kleinman, A., Das, V. and Lock, M. (eds) *Social Suffering.* University of California Press. Berkeley.

Fassin, D. (2001) The biopolitics of otherness: undocumented foreigners and racial discrimination in French public debate. *Anthropology Today* 17(1), 3–7.

Fassin, D. (2005) Compassion and repression: the moral economy of immigration policies in France. *Cultural Anthropology* 20(3), 362–387.

Fassin, D. and Naude, A.-J. (2004) Plumbism reinvented: childhood lead poisoning in France, 1985–1990. *American Journal of Public Health 1854–1863*, 94(11), 1854–1863.

Ferguson, D. and Horwood, L. (2003) Resilience to childhood adversity: results of a 21-year study. In Luthar, S. (ed.) *Resilience and Vulnerability: Adaptation in the Context of Childhood Adversities.* Cambridge University Press. Cambridge.

Fernando, S. (2005) Mental health services in the UK: lessons from transcultural psychiatry. In Ingleby, D. (ed.) *Forced Migration and Mental Health: Rethinking the Care of Refugees and Displaced Persons.* Springer. New York.

Fiddes, P. (1989) *Past Event and Present Salvation: The Christian Idea of Atonement.* Westminster John Knox Press. London.

Finch, N. (2005) Seeking asylum alone. In Andersson, H., Ascher, H., Bjornberg, U., Eastmund, M. and Mellander, L. (eds) *The Asylum Seeking Child in Europe.* Gothenburg University. Gothenburg.

Fink, J. (ed.) (2004) *Care: Personal Lives and Social Policy.* Open University Press. Milton Keynes.

Foster, G. (1965) Peasant society and the image of the limited good. *American Anthropologist* 67(2), 293–315.

Foucault, M. (1991) Governmentality. In Burchell, B., Gordon, G. and Miller, P. (eds) *The Foucault Effect: Studies in Governmentality.* University of Chicago Press. Chicago.

Frazer, N. (1997) *Justice Interruptus: Critical Reflections on the 'Postsocialist Condition'.* Routledge. New York.

Free, E. (2005) *Local Authority Support to Unaccompanied Asylum-seeking Young People. Changes since the Hillingdon Judgement (2003).* Save the Children England Programme.

Freud, A. and Burlingham, D. (1943) *War and Children.* Ernst Willard. New York.

Fukuyama, F. (1999) *Social capital and civil society.* Address to the International Monetary Fund 2nd Generation Conference.

Furedi, F. (2003) *Therapy Culture: Cultivating Vulnerability in an Uncertain Age.* Routledge. London.

Gardner, K. (2002) *Age, Narrative and Migration.* Oxford. Berg.

Ghorashi, H. (2005) Agents of change or passive victims: the impact of welfare states (the case of the Netherlands) on refugees. *Journal of Refugee Studies* 18(2), 181–198.

Giddens, A. (1984) *The Constitution of Society.* Polity Press. Cambridge.

Giddens, A. (1993) *New Rules of Sociological Method: A Positive Critique of Interpretative Sociologies.* 2nd Edition. Stanford University Press. Stanford, CA.

Gold, P. (2000) *Europe or Africa? A Contemporary Study of the Spanish North African Enclaves of Ceuta and Melilla.* Liverpool University Press. Liverpool.

Goldberg, D. and Huxley, P. (1994) *Common Mental Disorders: A Bio-Social Model.* Routledge. London.

Good, A. (2007) *Anthropology and Expertise in the Asylum Courts.* Routledge-Cavendish. Abingdon.

Goodwin, S. (1997) *Comparative Mental Health Policy: From Institutional to Community Care.* Sage. London.

Gramsci, A. (1971) *Selections from the Prison Notebooks.* Laurence and Wishart. London.

Gregory, D. (2004) *The Colonial Present.* Blackwell Publishing. Oxford.

Gunaratnam, Y. (2004) Skin matters: 'race' and care in the health services. In Fink, J. (ed.) *Care: Personal Lives and Social Policy.* Open University Press. Milton Keynes.

Hall, S. (1992) New ethnicities. In Donald, J. and Rattansi, A. *'Race', Culture and Difference.* Open University Press. Milton Keynes.

Hallberg, P. and Lund, J. (2005) The business of apocalypse: Robert Putnam and diversity. *Race and Class* 46(4), 53–67.

Halpern, D. (2005) *Social Capital.* Polity Press. Cambridge.

Hamilton, R., Anderson, A., Frater-Mathieson, K., Loewen, S. and Moore, D. (2006) *Interventions for Refugee Children in New Zealand Schools: Models, Methods and Best Practice.* Ministry of Education, New Zealand.

Handy, D. (1994) *Understanding Organisations.* 4th Edition. Penguin Books. London.

Hart, J. (2004) Beyond struggle and aid. Children's identities in a Palestinian refugee camp in Jordan. In Boyden, J. and de Berry, J. (eds) *Children and Youth on the Front Line.* Berghahn Books. New York.

Hart, R. (1992) *Children's Participation: From Tokenism to Citizenship.* UNESCO. Florence.

Harvey, D. (2005) *A Brief History of Neoliberalism.* Oxford University Press. Oxford.

Held, D., McGrew, A., Goldblatt, D. and Perraton, J. (1999) *Global Transformations: Politics, Economics and Culture.* Polity Press. Cambridge.

Heaton, J. (1999) The gaze and visibility of the carer. *Sociology of Health and Illness* 21(6), 759–777.

Her Majesty's Chief Inspector of Prisons (2004) *Report on a Full Announced Inspection of Dover Immigration Removal Centre.* Her Majesty's Chief Inspectorate of Prisons. London.

Hessle, M. (2005) *Asylum-seeking Children with Severe Withdrawal Behaviour – Status of Knowledge and Survey.* Statens Offentliga Utredningar. Stockholm.

HMSO (1989) *The Children Act 1989.* Crown Copyright. HMSO. London.

HMSO (2001a) *Select Committee on Home Affairs First Report 31st January 2001.* HMSO. London.

HMSO (2001b) *Border Controls.* Parliamentary Home Affairs report. HMSO. London.

Hobsbawm, E. (1994) *The Age of Extremes: The Short Twentieth Century 1914–1991.* Abacus. London.

Home Office (2000) Age disputes. *Policy Bulletin 33.* October 2000. Immigration and Nationality Directorate. London.

Home Office (2004) Press release, 2nd February. Home Office.

Home Office (2005) *Processing Applications from Children.* 3rd Edition. HMSO.

House of Commons (2002) *Hansard.* Volume 388, 9th July.

Human Rights and Equal Opportunity Commission (Australia) (2004) *A Last Resort? National Inquiry into Children in Immigration Detention.* Australian Government Publishing Service. Canberra.

Human Rights Watch (2002a) *Nowhere to Turn: State Abuses of Unaccompanied Migrant Children by Spain and Morocco.* Human Rights Watch. New York.

Human Rights Watch (2002b) *Spain and Morocco Abuse Child Migrants.* http://www.hrw.org/ press/2002/05/spain0507-testimony.htm, accessed 21st September 2006.

Human Rights Watch (2006) *Stemming the Flow: Abuses Against Migrants, Asylum Seekers and Refugees.* Report September 2006. Volume 18, No. 5(E).

Human Rights Without Frontiers (2003) *Annual Report: Belgium.* Human Rights Without Frontiers. Brussels.

Humphries, B. and Mynott, E. (2001) *Living your Life across Boundaries: Young Separated Refugees in Greater Manchester.* Save the Children. London.

Huntingdon, S. (1993) The clash of civilisations? *Foreign Affairs* 72(3), 22–49.

Ignatieff, M. (2001) *Human Rights as Politics and Idolatry.* Princeton University Press. Princeton.

Inda, J. (2006) *Targeting Immigrants: Government, Technology and Ethics.* Blackwell Publishing. Malden, MA.

Ingleby, D. (2005a) Meeting the needs of young asylum seekers: the role of creative activities. In Andersson, H., Ascher, H., Bjornberg, U., Eastmond, M. and Mellander, L. (eds) *The Asylum Seeking Child in Europe.* Gothenburg University. Gothenburg.

Ingleby, D. (ed.) (2005b) *Forced Migration and Mental Health: Rethinking the Care of Refugees and Displaced Persons.* Springer. New York.

Ingleby, D. and Watters, C. (2002) Refugee children at school: good practices in mental health and social care. *Education and Health* 20(3).

International Federation for Human Rights (2005) *Right to Asylum in Italy: Access to Procedures and Treatment of Asylum Seekers.* IFHR. Brussels.

James, A. and James, A. (2004) *Constructing Childhood: Theory, Policy and Social Practice.* Palgrave. Macmillan. Basingstoke.

James, A., Jenks, C. and Prout, A. (1998) *Theorising Childhood.* Polity Press. Cambridge.

Jones, L. (2004) *Then They Started Shooting: Growing up in Wartime Bosnia.* Harvard University Press. Cambridge, MA.

Kiecolt, G., Janice, K., Page, G., Marucha, P. and MacCallum, R. (1998) Psychological influences on surgical recovery: perspectives from psychoneuroimmunology. *American Psychologist* 53(11), 1209–1218.

Kingdon, J. (1984) *Bridging Research and Policy.* Harper Collins. New York.

Kleinman, A. (1977) Depression, somatisation and the new cross cultural psychiatry. *Social Science and Medicine* 11, 3–10.

Kleinman, A. (1988) *The Illness Narratives: Suffering, Healing and the Human Condition.* Basic Books. USA.

Kleinman, A., Das, V. and Lock, M. (1997) *Social Suffering.* University of California Press. Berkeley.

Knudsen, J. (1995) When trust is on trial: negotiating refugee narratives. In Valentine Daniel, E. and Knudsen, J. (eds) *Mistrusting Refugees.* University of California Press. Berkeley.

Kockel, U. (1999) *Borderline Cases: The Ethnic Frontiers of European Integration.* Liverpool University Press. Liverpool.

Korac, M. (2003) Integration and how we facilitate it: a comparative study of the settlement experiences of refugees in Italy and the Netherlands. *Sociology* 37(1), 51–68.

Kremer, P. (2002) Sangatte: a place of hope and despair. Red Cross–Red Crescent. *The magazine of the Red Cross and Red Crescent Movement.*

Kurtz, S. (1994) *All the Mothers Are One: Hindu India and the Cultural Reshaping of Psychoanalysis.* Columbia University Press. New York.

Kyambi, S. (2005) *Beyond Black and White: Mapping New Immigrant Communities.* Institute of Public Policy Research. London.

Laws, S., Harper, C. and Marcus, R. (2003) *Research for Development: A Practical Guide.* Save the Children. Sage. London.

Lewis, P. (2006) 500 children face forcible repatriation. *Guardian*, 18th August.

Liddicot (2003) Development of services for unaccompanied asylum seeking children. *Social Services Review Panel Report*, 6.

Lindstrom, C. (2002) *Report on the Situation of Refugees in Morocco: Findings of an Exploratory Study.* FMRS/American University of Cairo. Cairo.

Lipsky, M. (1980) *Street-Level Bureaucracy: Dilemmas of the Individual in Public Services.* Russell Sage Foundation. New York.

Local Government Act (1966) Her Majesty's Government.

London Boroughs of Hillingdon and Croydon (2004) *Practice Guidelines for Age Assessment of Young Unaccompanied Asylum Seekers*. London Boroughs of Hillingdon and Croydon.

Lukes, S. (2005) *Power: A Radical View*. Palgrave. Basingstoke.

Luthar, S. (ed.) (2003) *Resilience and Vulnerability: Adaptation in the Context of Childhood Adversities*. Cambridge University Press. Cambridge.

Lutterbeck, D. (2006) Policing migration in the Mediterranean. *Mediterranean Politics* 11(1), 59–82.

Lyon, M. (1993) Psychoneuroimmunology: the problem of the situatedness of illness and the conceptualisation of healing. *Culture, Medicine and Psychiatry* 17, 77–79.

Malkki, L. (1995a) *Purity and Exile: Violence, Memory and National Cosmology among Hutu Refugees in Tanzania*. University of Chicago Press. Chicago.

Malkki, L. (1995b) Refugees and exile: from 'refugee studies' to the national order of things. *American Review of Anthropology* 24, 495–523.

Mann, G. (2004) Separated children: care and support. In Boyden, J. and de Berry, J. (eds) *Children and Youth on the Front Line*. Berghahn Books. New York.

Martins, F. (2006) Personal communication.

Masten, A. and Powell, J. (2003) A resilience framework for research, policy and practice. In Luthar, S. (ed.) (2003) *Resilience and Vulnerability: Adaptation in the Context of Childhood Adversities*. Cambridge University Press. Cambridge.

McKeever, D., Shultz, J. and Swithern, S (2005) *Foreign Territory: The Internationalisation of EU Asylum Policy*. Oxfam Publications. Oxford.

Mead, M. (2001) *Coming of Age in Samoa*. Perennial Classics Edition. HarperCollins. New York.

Médecins Sans Frontières (2003) *International Activity Report 2002: Spain. Denouncing Refugee Detention Conditions*. MSF. Geneva.

Mels, C. and Derluyn, I. (2006) *Refugee Children and Adolescents and their Schools: Focus Groups with Parents in Belgium*. Gent University. Gent.

Milne, D. (1987) Problems and solutions in evaluation. In Milne, D. (ed.) *Evaluating Mental Health Practice: Methods and Applications*. Croom Helm. Beckenham.

M'Jid, N. (2005) *The situation of unaccompanied minors in Morocco*. Regional conference on migration of unaccompanied minors: acting in the best interests of the child. Council of Europe. Malaga.

Molano, A. (2005) *The Dispossessed: Chronicles of the Desterrados of Columbia*. Haymarket Books. Chicago.

Moorehead, C. (2005) *Human Cargo: A Journey Among Refugees*. Chatto and Windus. London.

Morris, L. (1998) Governing at a distance: the elaboration of controls in British immigration. *International Migration Review* 32(4), 949–973.

Moura, P. (2005) Dying to reach Europe. *Sign and Sight*, 13th October. www.signandsight.com, accessed 22nd April 2006.

Muecke, M. (1992) New paradigms for refugee health problems. *Social Science and Medicine* 35(4), 515–523.

Oloyede, O. (2002) A call for cultural sensitivity is not cultural relativism. *Mediche Anthropologie* 14(2), 297–302.

Ong, A. (1995) Making the biopolitical subject: Cambodian immigrants, refugee medicine and cultural citizenship in California. *Social Science and Medicine* 40(9), 1243–1257.

Ong, A. (2003) *Buddha is Hiding: Refugees, Citizenship, the New America.* University of California Press. Berkeley.

Owen, C. (2004) *Analysis of 2001 census data on numbers of black and mixed race children.* Working paper. Thomas Coram Research Unit. Institute of Education, University of London. London.

Page, B. (2006) *Race, Immigration and Identity in 2006 – The Big Picture.* Ipsos MORI Social Research Institute. London.

De Pauw, H. (2002) The disappearance of unaccompanied minors and minors victims of trafficking in human beings. April, p108. Child Focus. Brussels.

Pharos (2007) Pharos school prevention programmes for refugee and asylum seeking children. www.pharos.nl, accessed 7th March 2007.

Phillips, C. (2001) *Strangers in a Strange Land. Guardian,* 17th November.

Plummer, K. (2001) *Documents of Life: An Invitation to a Critical Humanism.* Sage. London.

Popkewitz, T. and Brennan, M. (1997) Restructuring of social and political theory in education: Foucault and a social epistemology of school practices. *Educational Theory* 47(3), 287–313.

Port of Dover police (2003) 2003 annual report. http://www.doverport.co.uk/library/pdf/police/POD%20Police%20Annual%20Report%202003.pdf, accessed 23rd June 2006.

Port of Zeebrugge (2006) www.zeebruggeport.be, accessed 12th August 2006.

Portes, A. (1998) Social capital: its origins and applications to modern sociology. *Annual Review of Sociology* 24, 1–24.

Pourgourides, C.K., Sashidharan, S.P. and Bracken, P.J. (1996) *A Second Exile: The Mental Health Implications of Detention of Asylum Seekers in the United Kingdom.* Northern Birmingham Mental Health Trust and University of Bradford.

Pred, A. (2000) *Even in Sweden: Racisms, Racialized Spaces, and the Popular Geographical Imagination.* California Studies in Critical Human Geography 8. University of California Press. Berkeley.

Pridmore, P. and Stephens, D. (2000) *Children as Partners for Health: A Critical Review of the Child-to-Child Approach.* Zed Books. London.

Puggioni, R. (2005) Refugees, institutional invisibility, and self-help strategies: evaluating Kurdish experience in Rome. *Journal of Refugee Studies* 18(3), 319–339.

Putnam, R. (2002) *Democracies in Flux: The Evolution of Social Capital in Contemporary Society.* Oxford University Press. Oxford.

Putnam, R. and Goss, K. (2002) Introduction. In Putnam, R. (ed) *Democracies in Flux: The Evolution of Social Capital in Contemporary Society.* Oxford University Press. Oxford.

Rack, P. (1982) *Race, Culture and Mental Disorder.* Tavistock. London.

Rapport, N. (2006) *In praise of displacement.* Keynote address at the Advanced Studies Institute on Refugees, Mental Health and Human Rights. McGill University. Montreal.

Red Cross (2004) *Guidelines from the Jesolo Conference on the EC Directive on minimum reception standards for asylum seekers.* Red Cross–EU. Brussels.

Red Cross (2006) *Final Report of the European Open Forum on Reception and Health Care of Asylum Seekers.* Austrian Red Cross, Red Cross–EU. Brussels.

Report of the Secretary General to the United Nations General Assembly on Protection and Assistance to Unaccompanied and Separated Refugee Children. 7th September 2001, (A/56/333).

Robben, A. and Suarez-Orozco, M. (2000) *Cultures Under Siege: Collective Violence and Trauma.* Cambridge University Press. Cambridge.

Rose, N. (1998) *Inventing Our Selves: Psychology, Power and Personhood.* Cambridge University Press. Cambridge.

Rose, N. (1999a) *Governing the Soul: The Shaping of the Private Self.* 2nd Edition. Free Association. London.

Rose, N. (1999b) *Powers of Freedom: Reframing Political Thought.* Cambridge University Press. Cambridge.

Rousseau, C., Drapeau, A., Lacroix, L., Bagilishya, D. and Heusch, N. (2005) Evaluation of a classroom program of creative expression workshops for refugee and immigrant children. *Journal of Child Psychology and Psychiatry* 46(2), 180–185.

Royal College of Paediatrics and Child Health (1999) *The Health of Refugee Children: Guidelines for Paediatricians.* London.

Rutter, J. (2003) *Supporting Refugee Children in 21st Century Britain: A Compendium of Essential Information.* Trentham Books. Stoke on Trent.

Rutter, J. (2006) *Refugee Children in the UK.* Open University Press. Maidenhead.

Ruuk, N. de (2002) *The Pharos School Prevention Programme Manual.* Final report of project for the European Commission (European Refugee Fund). University of Kent. Canterbury.

Said, E. (1978) *Orientalism: Western Conceptions of the Orient.* Penguin Books. London.

Said, E. (2001) *Reflections on Exile.* Granta Books. London.

Said, E. (2004) *Power, Politics and Culture.* Bloomsbury. London.

Sameroff, A., Gutman, L. and Peck, S. (2003) Adaptation among youths facing multiple risks: prospective research findings. In Luthar, S. (ed.) *Resilience and Vulnerability: Adaptation in the Context of Childhood Adversities.* Cambridge University Press. Cambridge.

Save the Children (2000) *Separated Children in Europe Programme.* Statement of Good Practice, 2nd edition. October.

Scheper-Hughes, N. (1992) *Death Without Weeping: The Violence of Everyday Life in Brazil.* University of California Press. Berkeley.

Scheper-Hughes, N. and Sargent, C. (1998) *Small Wars: The Cultural Politics of Childhood.* University of California Press. Berkeley.

Schierup, C-U., Hansen, P. and Castles, S. (2006) *Migration, Citizenship, and the European Welfare State: A European Dilemma.* Oxford University Press. Oxford.

Scott, T., Short, E., Singer, L., Russ, S. and Minnes, S. (2006) Psychometric properties of the Dominic interactive assessment: a computerised self-report for children. *Assessment* 13(1), 16–26.

Sen, A. (1999) *Development as Freedom.* Oxford University Press. Oxford.

Sen, A. (2006) *Identity and Violence: The Illusion of Destiny.* Allen Lane. London.

Sennett, R. (2006) Preface. In Buonfino, A. and Mulgan, G. (eds) *Porcupines in Winter: The Pleasures and Pains of Living Together in Modern Britain.* The Young Foundation. London.

Silove, D., Steel, Z. and Watters, C. (2000) Policies of deterrence and the mental health of asylum seekers. *Journal of the American Medical Association* 284(5), 604–611.

Silove, D., Steel, Z., McGorry, P. and Dobny, J. (1999) Problems Tamil asylum seekers encounter in accessing health and welfare services in Australia. *Social Science and Medicine* 49, 951–956.

Simpson, L. (2006) *The place of abode of terrorist suspects.* Working paper. Cathie Marsh Centre for Census and Survey Research, Manchester University. Manchester.

Singer, P. (2006) *Children at War.* University of California Press. Berkeley.

Smith, T. (2005) *Promoting inclusion for unaccompanied young asylum seekers and immigrants – a duty of justice and care. A report of a two year transnational project involving government, local authorities NGOs and young asylum seekers.* European Social Network.

Social Inclusion Board (2003) *Everyone's Responsibility: Reducing Homelessness in South Australia.* Department of the Premier and Cabinet. Government of South Australia.

Stainton Rogers, W. (2001) Constructing childhood, constructing child concern. In Foley, P., Roche, J. and Tucker, S. (eds) *Children in Society: Contemporary Theory, Policy and Practice.* Open University Press. Milton Keynes.

Summerfield, D. (1999) A critique of seven assumptions behind psychological trauma programmes in war affected areas. *Social Science and Medicine* 48, 1449–1462.

Summerfield, D. (2005) 'My whole body is sick...my life is not good'. A Rwandan asylum seeker attends a psychiatric clinic in London. In Ingleby, D. (ed.) *Forced Migration and Mental Health: Rethinking the Care of Refugees and Displaced Persons.* Springer. New York.

Szalacha, L., Erkut, S., Coll, C., Fields, J., Alarcon, O. and Ceder, I. (2003) Perceived discrimination and resilience. In Luthar, S. (ed.) *Resilience and Vulnerability: Adaptation in the Context of Childhood Adversities.* Cambridge University Press. Cambridge.

Taussig, M. (2006) *Walter Benjamin's Grave.* University of Chicago Press. Chicago.

Thompson, E.P. (1971) The moral economy of the English crowd in the eighteenth century. *Past and Present* 50, 76–136.

Tremlett, G. (2005) Spain heightens fence at African enclave. *Guardian*, 22nd September.

Tremlett, G. (2006) Spain steps up patrols as 1,000 migrants die during desperate quest for Europe. *Guardian*, 23rd March.

Turton, D. (2003) *Refugees, forced settlers and 'other forced migrants': Towards a unitary study of forced migration: New issues in refugee research.* Working paper 94. UNHCR. Geneva.

UN (1989) Convention on the Rights of the Child.

UN (2005) UN Committee on the Rights of the Child, report on Sweden 30th March 2005. Office of the High Commissioner for Human Rights.

UNESCO (1999) *Education for All Thematic Study: Education in Situations of Emergency and Crisis.* Emergency Educational Assistance Unit. Paris.

UNHCR (1992a) *Handbook on Procedures and Criteria for Determining Refugee Status.* UNHCR. Geneva.

UNHCR (1992b) *Conclusions and Decisions 31 (d) 1992.* UNHCR. Geneva.

UNHCR (1994) *Refugee Children – Guidelines on Protection and Care.* UNHCR. Geneva.

UNHCR (2001) *Women, Children and Older Refugees.* UNHCR. Geneva.

UNHCR (2004) *Trends in Unaccompanied and Separated Children Seeking Asylum in Industrialised Countries, 2001–2003.* United Nations High Commissioner for Refugees. Geneva.

UNHCR (2005) Z Obcej Ziemi. No 23. http://www.unhcr.pl/english/newsletter/23/dostep.php, accessed 29th October 2006.

UNHCR (2006a) *2005 Global Refugee Trends: Statistical Overview of Populations of Refugees, Asylum Seekers, Internally Displaced Persons, Stateless Persons, and other Persons of Concern to UNHCR.* UNHCR. Geneva.

UNHCR (2006b) *The State of the World's Refugees: Human Displacement in the New Millennium.* Oxford University Press. Oxford.

UNHCR (2006c) *Refugees by Numbers* 2006 Edition. www.unhcr.org, accessed 21st April 2006.

UNHCR (2007) *Asylum Levels and Trends in Industrialised Countries, 2006*. Division of Operational Services. UNHCR. Geneva.

Valentine Daniel, E. and Knudsen, J. (eds) (1995) *Mistrusting Refugees*. University of California Press. Berkeley.

Van Hear, N. (2006) 'I went as far as my money would take me': conflict, forced migration and class. In Crepeau, F., Nakache, D., Collyer, M. *et al.* (eds) *Forced Migration and Global Processes*. Lexington Books. Maryland.

Vasta, E. (2006) *From ethnic minorities to ethnic majority policy: changing identities and the shift to assimilation in the Netherlands*. Working paper 26. COMPAS. University of Oxford. Oxford.

Verdirame, G. and Harrell-Bond, B. (2005) *Rights in Exile: Janus-Faced Humanitarianism*. Studies in Forced Migration 17. Berghahn Books. New York.

Wacquant, L. (1992) *The Structure and Logic of Bourdieu's Sociology in Bourdieu and Wacquant: An Invitation to Reflexive Sociology*. Polity Press. Cambridge.

Wade, J., Mitchell, F. and Baylis, G. (2005) *Unaccompanied Asylum Seeking Children: The Response of Social Work Services*. British Association for Adoption and Fostering. London.

Walkerdine, V. (2006) *Negotiating identity, disadvantage and dislocation*. Paper presented at the ESRC Identities and Social Action Conference. Birmingham.

Ward, L. (2006) Free English lessons for adult asylum seekers to be axed. *Guardian*, 28th December.

Watters, C. (1996a) Inequalities in mental health: the inner city mental health project. *Journal of Community and Applied Psychology* 6, 383–394.

Watters, C. (1996b) Representations of Asians in British psychiatry. In C. Samson and N. South (eds) *Conflict and Consensus in Social Policy, Racism, Citizenship and the Environment*, (pp.88–105). Explorations in Sociology 44. British Sociological Association. Macmillan. London.

Watters, C. (2001a) Emerging paradigms in the mental health care of refugees. *Social Science and Medicine* 52, 1709–1718.

Watters, C. (2001b) Avenues of access and the moral economy of legitimacy. *Anthropology Today* 17(2), 22–23.

Watters, C. (2001c) Author's fieldwork note. Unpublished.

Watters, C. (2002a) *Asylum Seekers and Mental Health Care in the UK*. Refugee Council. London.

Watters, C. (2002b) Migration and mental health care in Europe: report on a preliminary mapping exercise. *Journal of Ethnic and Migration Studies* 28, 153–172.

Watters, C. (2003) Author's fieldwork note. Unpublished.

Watters, C. (2006) Personal communication – interview with a shipping police officer, 3rd February.

Watters, C. (2007) Reflections on policy responses to migrants in Europe: the Netherlands and Sweden. In Wetherall, M. (ed.) (2007) *Identities and Social Action Programme Submission to the Commission on Integration and Cohesion*. Economic and Social Research Council Programme on Identities and Social Action. Unpublished.

Watters, C. and Ingleby, D. (2004) Locations of care: meeting the mental health and social care needs of refugees in Europe. *International Journal of Law and Psychiatry* 27, 549–570.

Watters, C., Ingleby, D., Bernal, M., De Freitas, C., de Ruuk, N., Van Leeuwen, M. and Venkatesan, S. (2003) *Good Practices in Mental Health and Social Care for Asylum Seekers and Refugees*. Final report of project for the European Commission (European Refugee Fund). University of Kent. Canterbury.

Weiss, T. and Korn, D. (2006) *Internal Displacement: Conceptualisation and its Consequences*. Global Institutions. Routledge. Abingdon.

Wetherall, M. (2007) *Identities and Social Action Programme Submission to the Commission on Integration and Cohesion*. Economic and Social Research Council Programme on Identities and Social Action. Unpublished.

Wheeler, S. (2002) Belgium's 'missing' migrant children. BBC News, 18th June. http://news.bbc.co.uk/1/hi/world/europe/2051904.stm, accessed 22 August 2007.

Whimster, S. (2004) *The Essential Weber: A Reader*. Routledge. London.

Williams, L. (2006) *Refugees, Transnationalism and New Community Spaces*. Unpublished PhD Thesis. University of Kent. Canterbury.

Wood, T. (2004) The case for Chechnya. *New Left Review* 30, 5–36.

World Health Organization (1996) *The Mental Health of Refugees*. WHO. Geneva.

Yaghmaian, B. (2005) *Embracing the Infidel: Stories of Muslim Migrants on the Journey West*. Delacorte Press. New York.

Young, A. (1995) *The Harmony of Illusions: Inventing Post-Traumatic Stress Disorder*. Princeton University Press. Princeton.

Zapatero, L. (2005) Europe is the Answer. *Guardian*, 26th October 2006.

Zolberg, A. (1989) The next waves: migration theory for a changing world. *International Migration Review* 23(3), 403–430.

Zolberg, A., Suhrke, A. and Aguayo, S. (1989) *Escape From Violence: Conflict and the Refugee Crisis in the Developing World*. Oxford University Press. Oxford.

Index

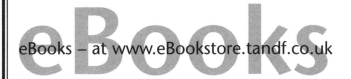

Smith, T. (2005) *Promoting inclusion for unaccompanied young asylum seekers and immigrants – a duty of justice and care. A report of a two year transnational project involving government, local authorities NGOs and young asylum seekers.* European Social Network.

Social Inclusion Board (2003) *Everyone's Responsibility: Reducing Homelessness in South Australia.* Department of the Premier and Cabinet. Government of South Australia.

Stainton Rogers, W. (2001) Constructing childhood, constructing child concern. In Foley, P., Roche, J. and Tucker, S. (eds) *Children in Society: Contemporary Theory, Policy and Practice.* Open University Press. Milton Keynes.

Summerfield, D. (1999) A critique of seven assumptions behind psychological trauma programmes in war affected areas. *Social Science and Medicine* 48, 1449–1462.

Summerfield, D. (2005) 'My whole body is sick...my life is not good'. A Rwandan asylum seeker attends a psychiatric clinic in London. In Ingleby, D. (ed.) *Forced Migration and Mental Health: Rethinking the Care of Refugees and Displaced Persons.* Springer. New York.

Szalacha, L., Erkut, S., Coll, C., Fields, J., Alarcon, O. and Ceder, I. (2003) Perceived discrimination and resilience. In Luthar, S. (ed.) *Resilience and Vulnerability: Adaptation in the Context of Childhood Adversities.* Cambridge University Press. Cambridge.

Taussig, M. (2006) *Walter Benjamin's Grave.* University of Chicago Press. Chicago.

Thompson, E.P. (1971) The moral economy of the English crowd in the eighteenth century. *Past and Present* 50, 76–136.

Tremlett, G. (2005) Spain heightens fence at African enclave. *Guardian*, 22nd September.

Tremlett, G. (2006) Spain steps up patrols as 1,000 migrants die during desperate quest for Europe. *Guardian*, 23rd March.

Turton, D. (2003) *Refugees, forced settlers and 'other forced migrants': Towards a unitary study of forced migration: New issues in refugee research.* Working paper 94. UNHCR. Geneva.

UN (1989) Convention on the Rights of the Child.

UN (2005) UN Committee on the Rights of the Child, report on Sweden 30th March 2005. Office of the High Commissioner for Human Rights.

UNESCO (1999) *Education for All Thematic Study: Education in Situations of Emergency and Crisis.* Emergency Educational Assistance Unit. Paris.

UNHCR (1992a) *Handbook on Procedures and Criteria for Determining Refugee Status.* UNHCR. Geneva.

UNHCR (1992b) *Conclusions and Decisions 31 (d) 1992.* UNHCR. Geneva.

UNHCR (1994) *Refugee Children – Guidelines on Protection and Care.* UNHCR. Geneva.

UNHCR (2001) *Women, Children and Older Refugees.* UNHCR. Geneva.

UNHCR (2004) *Trends in Unaccompanied and Separated Children Seeking Asylum in Industrialised Countries, 2001–2003.* United Nations High Commissioner for Refugees. Geneva.

UNHCR (2005) Z Obcej Ziemi. No 23. http://www.unhcr.pl/english/newsletter/23/dostep.php, accessed 29th October 2006.

UNHCR (2006a) *2005 Global Refugee Trends: Statistical Overview of Populations of Refugees, Asylum Seekers, Internally Displaced Persons, Stateless Persons, and other Persons of Concern to UNHCR.* UNHCR. Geneva.

UNHCR (2006b) *The State of the World's Refugees: Human Displacement in the New Millennium.* Oxford University Press. Oxford.

UNHCR (2006c) *Refugees by Numbers* 2006 Edition. www.unhcr.org, accessed 21st April 2006.

UNHCR (2007) *Asylum Levels and Trends in Industrialised Countries, 2006.* Division of Operational Services. UNHCR. Geneva.

Valentine Daniel, E. and Knudsen, J. (eds) (1995) *Mistrusting Refugees.* University of California Press. Berkeley.

Van Hear, N. (2006) 'I went as far as my money would take me': conflict, forced migration and class. In Crepeau, F., Nakache, D., Collyer, M. *et al.* (eds) *Forced Migration and Global Processes.* Lexington Books. Maryland.

Vasta, E. (2006) *From ethnic minorities to ethnic majority policy: changing identities and the shift to assimilation in the Netherlands.* Working paper 26. COMPAS. University of Oxford. Oxford.

Verdirame, G. and Harrell-Bond, B. (2005) *Rights in Exile: Janus-Faced Humanitarianism.* Studies in Forced Migration 17. Berghahn Books. New York.

Wacquant, L. (1992) *The Structure and Logic of Bourdieu's Sociology in Bourdieu and Wacquant: An Invitation to Reflexive Sociology.* Polity Press. Cambridge.

Wade, J., Mitchell, F. and Baylis, G. (2005) *Unaccompanied Asylum Seeking Children: The Response of Social Work Services.* British Association for Adoption and Fostering. London.

Walkerdine, V. (2006) *Negotiating identity, disadvantage and dislocation.* Paper presented at the ESRC Identities and Social Action Conference. Birmingham.

Ward, L. (2006) Free English lessons for adult asylum seekers to be axed. *Guardian*, 28th December.

Watters, C. (1996a) Inequalities in mental health: the inner city mental health project. *Journal of Community and Applied Psychology* 6, 383–394.

Watters, C. (1996b) Representations of Asians in British psychiatry. In C. Samson and N. South (eds) *Conflict and Consensus in Social Policy, Racism, Citizenship and the Environment*, (pp.88–105). Explorations in Sociology 44. British Sociological Association. Macmillan. London.

Watters, C. (2001a) Emerging paradigms in the mental health care of refugees. *Social Science and Medicine* 52, 1709–1718.

Watters, C. (2001b) Avenues of access and the moral economy of legitimacy. *Anthropology Today* 17(2), 22–23.

Watters, C. (2001c) Author's fieldwork note. Unpublished.

Watters, C. (2002a) *Asylum Seekers and Mental Health Care in the UK.* Refugee Council. London.

Watters, C. (2002b) Migration and mental health care in Europe: report on a preliminary mapping exercise. *Journal of Ethnic and Migration Studies* 28, 153–172.

Watters, C. (2003) Author's fieldwork note. Unpublished.

Watters, C. (2006) Personal communication – interview with a shipping police officer, 3rd February.

Watters, C. (2007) Reflections on policy responses to migrants in Europe: the Netherlands and Sweden. In Wetherall, M. (ed.) (2007) *Identities and Social Action Programme Submission to the Commission on Integration and Cohesion.* Economic and Social Research Council Programme on Identities and Social Action. Unpublished.

Watters, C. and Ingleby, D. (2004) Locations of care: meeting the mental health and social care needs of refugees in Europe. *International Journal of Law and Psychiatry* 27, 549–570.

Watters, C., Ingleby, D., Bernal, M., De Freitas, C., de Ruuk, N., Van Leeuwen, M. and Venkatesan, S. (2003) *Good Practices in Mental Health and Social Care for Asylum Seekers and Refugees.* Final report of project for the European Commission (European Refugee Fund). University of Kent. Canterbury.

Weiss, T. and Korn, D. (2006) *Internal Displacement: Conceptualisation and its Consequences.* Global Institutions. Routledge. Abingdon.

Wetherall, M. (2007) *Identities and Social Action Programme Submission to the Commission on Integration and Cohesion.* Economic and Social Research Council Programme on Identities and Social Action. Unpublished.

Wheeler, S. (2002) Belgium's 'missing' migrant children. BBC News, 18th June. http://news.bbc.co.uk/1/hi/world/europe/2051904.stm, accessed 22 August 2007.

Whimster, S. (2004) *The Essential Weber: A Reader.* Routledge. London.

Williams, L. (2006) *Refugees, Transnationalism and New Community Spaces.* Unpublished PhD Thesis. University of Kent. Canterbury.

Wood, T. (2004) The case for Chechnya. *New Left Review* 30, 5–36.

World Health Organization (1996) *The Mental Health of Refugees.* WHO. Geneva.

Yaghmaian, B. (2005) *Embracing the Infidel: Stories of Muslim Migrants on the Journey West.* Delacorte Press. New York.

Young, A. (1995) *The Harmony of Illusions: Inventing Post-Traumatic Stress Disorder.* Princeton University Press. Princeton.

Zapatero, L. (2005) Europe is the Answer. *Guardian*, 26th October 2006.

Zolberg, A. (1989) The next waves: migration theory for a changing world. *International Migration Review* 23(3), 403–430.

Zolberg, A., Suhrke, A. and Aguayo, S. (1989) *Escape From Violence: Conflict and the Refugee Crisis in the Developing World.* Oxford University Press. Oxford.